OXFORD MEDICAL PUBLICATIONS

Emergencies in Primary Care

Emergencies in Primary Care

Edited by

Chantal Simon
GP, and MRC Health Service Research Fellow,
Department of Primary Medical Care, Southampton
University Medical School and Tottan, Southampton

Karen O'Reilly
GP, Bishops Waltham

John Buckmaster
GP, Isle of South Uist, Western Isles

Robin Proctor
GP, Hampshire

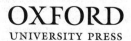

OXFORD
UNIVERSITY PRESS

OXFORD
UNIVERSITY PRESS

Great Clarendon Street, Oxford OX2 6DP

Oxford University Press is a department of the University of Oxford.
It furthers the University's objective of excellence in research, scholarship,
and education by publishing worldwide in

Oxford New York

Auckland Cape Town Dar es Salaam Hong Kong Karachi
Kuala Lumpur Madrid Melbourne Mexico City Nairobi
New Delhi Shanghai Taipei Toronto

With offices in

Argentina Austria Brazil Chile Czech Republic France Greece
Guatemala Hungary Italy Japan Poland Portugal Singapore
South Korea Switzerland Thailand Turkey Ukraine Vietnam

Oxford is a registered trade mark of Oxford University Press
in the UK and in certain other countries

Published in the United States
by Oxford University Press Inc., New York

British Library Cataloguing in Publication Data

Data available

Library of Congress Cataloging in Publication Data

Data available

Typeset by Newgen Imaging Systems (P) Ltd., Chennai, India
Printed in China
on acid-free paper by
C&C offset printing Co., Ltd

ISBN 978–0–19–857068–4

10 9 8 7 6

Acknowledgements

This book would not have come into being without the support and drive of Fiona Goodgame, Chris Reid, Angela Butterworth and the rest of the team at Oxford University Press.

We would like to thank Anna Wilson for writing the section on child protection used within this book. We would also like to thank the authors of the *Oxford Handbook of General Practice*, and the authors of the Oxford General Practice Library—Hazel Everitt, Chantal Simon, Tony Kendrick, Richard Newsom, Richard Davies, Will Bolland, Max Watson, Karen O'Reilly, Nick Dunn, Jeannette Lynch, Francoise van Dorp, Carrie Sadler and Jo White—for allowing us to reproduce material within this volume.

Any text covering such a large range of clinical topics is hard to review, and we sincerely thank all our GP and expert reviewers for their attentiveness to detail and helpful comments when reviewing this text: Ian Wright, Anna Wilson, Zoë Crosby, Judith Harvey, Liz Oliver, David Hargreaves, Simon Crawford, Karen Brackley, Sue Connolly, Meme Wijesinghe, Malcolm Maclean, and Lesley Boyd.

Most of all we would like to thank our families for their patience and tolerance over the time this book has been in the making.

KOR
RP
JB
CS

Contents

Abbreviations

⚠	Warning
❶	Note
☎	Telephone number
💾	Website
📖	Cross reference to
±	With or without
↑	Increased/increasing
↓	Decreased/decreasing
→	Leading to
°	Degrees
1°	Primary
2°	Secondary
♂	Male
♀	Female
≈	Approximately equal
~	Approximately
%	Percent(age)
≥	Greater than or equal to
≤	Less than or equal to
>	Greater than
<	Less than
+ve	Positive
−ve	Negative
°	Degrees
C	Cochrane review
G	Guideline from major guideline producing body
N	NICE guidance
R	Randomized controlled trial in major journal
S	Systematic review in major journal
ND	Notifiable disease
β	Beta
A&E	Accident and Emergency
AED	Automated external defibrillator
AF	Atrial fibrillation
AIDS	Acquired immune deficiency syndrome
ALS	Advanced life support

ASO	Antistreptolysin titre
AV	Atrio-ventricular
A-V	Arteriovenous
bd	Twice daily
BHF	British Heart Foundation
BLS	Basic life support
BM	Blood glucose using reagent strip
BMA	British Medical Association
BMI	Body mass index
BMJ	British Medical Journal
BNF	British National Formulary
BP	Blood pressure
bpm	Beats per minute
BTS	British Thoracic Society
C	Centigrade
C_{1-8}	Cervical nerve roots
Ca^{2+}	Calcium
CAH	Congenital adrenal hyperplasia
CF	Cystic fibrosis
Cl^-	Chloride
cm	Centimetre(s)
CMV	Cytomegalovirus
CNS	Central nervous system
CO_2	Carbon dioxide
COC	Combined oral contraceptive
CPR	Cardiopulmonary resuscitation
Cr	Creatinine
CRP	C-reactive protein
CSF	Cerebrospinal fluid
CSM	Committee on Safety of Medicines
CT	Computerized tomography
CVD	Cardiovascular disease
CXR	Chest X-ray
d	Day(s)
DC	Direct current
dL	Decilitre
DLA	Disability Living Allowance
DM	Diabetes mellitus
DoH	Department of Health
DSH	Deliberate self-harm
DTB	Drugs and Therapeutic Bulletin
DWP	Department of Work and Pensions

EBV	Epstein–Barr virus
Echo	Echocardiogram
ECG	Electrocardiograph
EEG	Electro-encephalogram
e.g.	For example
eGFR	Estimated glomerular filtration rate
ENT	Ear, nose and throat
ESR	Erythrocyte sedimentation rate
ESRF	End-stage renal failure
etc.	Et cetera
F	Fahrenheit
FBAO	Foreign body airways obstruction
FBC	Full blood count
FEV_1	Forced expiratory volume in one second
FH	Family history
FVC	Forced vital capacity
g	grams
GA	General anaesthetic
GBS	Group B streptococcus
GI	gastrointestinal
GMC	General Medical Council
GMS	General Medical Services
GnRH	Gonadotrophin releasing hormone
GORD	Gastro-oesophageal reflux disease
Gp.	Group
GP	General practitioner
h	Hour(s)
Hb	Haemoglobin
HCV	Hepatitis C virus
HIV	Human immunodeficiency virus
HOCM	Hypertrophic obstructive cardiomyopathy
HSV	Herpes simplex virus
ICP	Intracranial pressure
Ig	Immunoglobulin
IM	Intramuscular
IO	Intraosseous
INR	International normalization ratio
IT	Information technology
IUCD	Intrauterine contraceptive device
IUGR	Intrauterine growth retardation
IUS	Intrauterine system
IV	Intravenous

J	Joules
JVP	Jugular venous pressure
K^+	Potassium
kg	Kilogram(s)
l	Litre(s)
L	Left
LABA	Long acting beta agonist
LFT	Liver function test
LMP	Last menstrual period
LMWH	Low molecular weight heparin
LN	Lymph node
LOC	Loss of consciousness
LRTI	Lower respiratory tract infection
LSCS	Lower segment Caesarean Section
LTOT	Long term oxygen therapy
LVF	Left ventricular failure
m	Metres
mcgm	Micrograms
M,C&S	Microscopy, culture and sensitivity
MCUG	Micturating cysto-urethrogram
MCV	Mean cell volume
MDI	Metered dose inhaler
mg	Milligrams
MHRA	Medicines & Healthcare Products Regulatory Agency
MI	Myocardial infarct
min	Minutes
ml	Millilitres
mmHg	Millimetres of mercury
mmol	Millimole
MMR	Measles, mumps and rubella
mo	Month(s)
MRSA	Methicillin resistant Staphylococcus aureus
MSU	Mid-stream urine
Na^+	Sodium
NAI	Non-accidental injury
NHS	National Health Service
NICE	National Institute for Clinical Excellence
nmol	Nanomoles
NNT	Number needed to treat
NSAID	Non-steroidal anti-inflammatory drug
NSF	National Service Framework
O_2	Oxygen

od	Once daily
OM	Otitis media
OOH	Out of hours
OTC	Over the counter
OUP	Oxford University Press
p.	Page number
P.	Plasmodium
PALS	Paediatric advanced life support
PBLS	Paediatric basic life support
PCO	Primary Care Organization
PCOS	Polycystic ovarian syndrome
PDA	Patent ductus arteriosus
PE	Pulmonary embolus
PEFR	Peak expiratory flow rate
PFBAO	Paediatric foreign body airways obstruction
Physio	Physiotherapy
PID	Pelvic inflammatory disease
PIP	Proximal interphalangeal joint
PMH	Past medical history
PMS	Personal Medical Services
po	Oral
prn	As needed
PTSD	Post-traumatic stress disorder
qds	Four times daily
QOF	Quality and outcomes framework
R	Right
RA	Rheumatoid arthritis
RCGP	Royal College of General Practitioners
RCN	Royal College of Nursing
RICE	rest, ice, compression, elevation
RSV	Respiratory syncytial virus
s or sec	Second (s)
S.	Streptococcus
SAH	Subarachnoid haemorrhage
SBE	Subacute bacterial endocarditis
s/cut	Subcutaneous
SIGN	Scottish Intercollegiate Guidelines Network
SOL	Space occupying lesion
SLE	Systemic lupus erythematosus
SPF	Sun-protection factor
Staph.	Staphylococcus
STD	Sexually transmitted disease

Strep.	Streptococcus
SVT	Supraventricular tachycardia
TB	Tuberculosis
Td	Tetanus and low dose diphtheria vaccine
tds	Three times a day
TFTs	Thyroid function tests
TSH	Thyroid stimulating hormone
u	Units
U&E	Urea and electrolytes
UC	Ulcerative colitis
UK	United Kingdom
URTI	Upper respiratory tract infection
USS	Ultrasound scan
UTI	Urinary tract infection
VF	Ventricular fibrillation
VT	Ventricular tachycardia
VZ	Varicella zoster
WCC	White cell count
WHO	World Health Organization
wk	Week(s)
WPW	Wolff–Parkinson–White syndrome
y	Year(s)

Introduction

Introduction

Emergencies can present to primary care at any time or in any place. In the community, conditions are often not ideal (e.g. patient on the floor, poor lighting, numerous layers of clothing) and support may not be immediately available. Management includes recognition of emergencies, their immediate care and any follow-up required. That can be both challenging and frightening. Good organization, teamwork, communication and situational awareness are vital.

In the last 10 years, the face of primary care in the UK has changed. Emergencies are now managed by a large range of medical staff ranging from GPs, through specialist nurses to paramedics. Although written for GPs, this book is designed as a brief guide to good practice for anyone managing primary care emergencies in the community.

Training: training required to manage primary care emergencies varies according to the health professional's role and level of back up available.

GPs in training: The Committee of Postgraduate General Practice Education Directors (COGPED) has stated that GP Registrars should continue to obtain experience in out-of-hours (OOH) care irrespective of whether their trainer has opted out of providing OOH care. They defined 6 core competencies (Box 1.1), which the RCGP later incorporated into their Curriculum Statement on 'Care of Acutely Ill People'.

Resuscitation skills: training and practice are necessary to acquire skill in resuscitation techniques. Resuscitation skills decline rapidly and updates and retraining using manikins are necessary every 6–12 mo to maintain adequate skill levels. Level of skill needed by different members of the primary health care team differs according to the individual's role:
- All those in direct contact with patients should be trained in basic life support (BLS) and related resuscitation skills, e.g. the recovery position
- Doctors, nurses and other paramedical workers (e.g. physiotherapists) should be able to use an automatic external defibrillator (AED). Other personnel (e.g. receptionists) may also be trained to use an AED.

❶ Practices are rewarded in the QOF (Education Indicators 1 and 5) for providing basic life support training to practice-employed staff.

Box 1.1 The 6 'generic competencies'

1. Ability to manage common medical, surgical and psychiatric emergencies in the OOH setting
2. Understanding of the organizational aspects of NHS OOH hours care
3. Ability to make appropriate referrals to hospitals and other professionals in the OOH setting
4. Demonstration of communication skills required for OOH care
5. Individual personal time and stress management
6. Maintenance of personal security and awareness and management of the security risks to others

Box 1.2 Knowledge base required for the GP Curriculum

Symptoms
- *Cardiovascular*—chest pain, haemorrhage, shock
- *Respiratory*—wheeze, breathlessness, stridor, choking
- *Central nervous system*—convulsions, ↓ conscious level, confusion
- *Mental health*—threatened self-harm, delusional states, violent patients
- *Severe pain*

Common and/or important conditions
- Shock (including no cardiac output), acute coronary syndromes, haemorrhage (revealed/concealed), ischaemia, pulmonary embolism, asthma
- Dangerous diagnoses (💭 p.4)
- Common problems that may be expected with certain practice activities: anaphylaxis after immunization, local anaesthetic toxicity and vaso-vagal attacks (e.g. with minor surgery or IUCD insertion)
- Parasuicide and suicide attempts

Investigation—blood glucose.

❶ Other investigations are rare in primary care because acutely ill patients needing investigation are usually referred to secondary care.

Treatment—pre-hospital management of convulsions and acute dyspnoea.

Emergency care
- The 'ABC' principles in initial management
- Appreciate response time required to optimize outcome
- Understand organizational aspects of NHS out of hours care
- Understand importance of maintaining personal security and awareness and management of the security risks to others

Resources
- Appropriate use of emergency services—including logistics of how to obtain an ambulance/paramedic crew
- Familiarity with available equipment in own car/bag and that carried by emergency services
- Selection and maintenance of appropriate equipment and un-expired drugs that should be carried by GPs
- Being able to organize/lead a response when required, which may include participation by staff, members of the public or qualified responders
- Knowledge of training required for practice staff and others as a team in the appropriate responses to an acutely ill person

Prevention
- Advice to patients on prevention; e.g. with a patient with known heart disease, advice on how to manage ischaemic pain, including use of GTN, aspirin and appropriate first-line use of paramedic ambulance

Dangerous diagnoses: in primary care, if a potentially life-threatening diagnosis is suspected, act as if the diagnosis was certain, and refer immediately to secondary care (Box 1.3). It is better to be wrong and appear over cautious, than miss a treatable condition that might otherwise be fatal. Problems occur where a doctor has correctly suspected that diagnosis, recorded it, but then not acted on the possibility.

Performance management

Significant event audit: recognized methodology for reflecting on important events in a practice. Many primary care emergencies are suitable topics for significant event audit. Practices undertaking significant event audit are eligible for quality points (Education Indicators 2 and 7). Discussion of specific events can:

- identify learning objectives *and*
- provoke emotions that can be harnessed to achieve change.

For it to be effective, significant event audit must be practised in a culture that avoids blame and involves all disciplines. There are 3 steps:

- *Decide on a topic and plan a meeting.* A list of suitable events can be made for an individual practice or a pre-formed list of suitable events is available from the RCGP (Significant Event Auditing: Occasional Paper 70, 1995).
- At the end of the discussion, *come to a decision* about the case, e.g. well managed, need change in procedure, etc.
- *Prepare a report.* The 2 acceptable formats for laying out these reports are described in Box 1.4.

Resuscitation attempts: accurate records of all resuscitation attempts and electronic data stored by most AEDs during a resuscitation attempt should be kept for audit, training and medico-legal reasons. The responsibility for this rests with the most senior member of the practice team involved. Process and outcome of all resuscitation attempts should be audited—at practice and PCO level—to allow deficiencies to be addressed, and examples of good practice to be shared.

Essential reading

RCGP Care of acutely ill people—Curriculum Statement 7 (2006) ▣ www.rcgp.org.uk

Resuscitation Council (UK) Cardiopulmonary resuscitation guidance for clinical practice and training in Primary Care (2005) ▣ www.resus.org.uk

Box 1.3 Dangerous diagnoses

- Myocardial infarction
- Pulmonary embolus
- Subarachnoid haemorrhage
- Appendicitis
- Limb ischaemia
- Intestinal obstruction or perforation
- Meningitis
- Aneurysms
- Ectopic pregnancy
- Acute psychosis/mania
- Visual problems that could lead to blindness including retinal detachment and haemorrhage as well as systemic disease such as temporal arteritis, which if not recognized has serious complications.

Box 1.4 Methods of reporting significant event audits

Reporting method 1

- *Description of event*—this should be brief and can be in note form.
- *Learning outcome*—this should describe the aspects that were of high standard and those that could be improved. Where appropriate it should include why the event occurred.
- *Action plan*—the decision(s) taken needs to be contained in the report. The reasons for these decisions should be described together with any other lessons learned from the discussion.

Reporting method 2

- What happened?
- Why did it happen?
- Was insight demonstrated?
- Was change implemented?

Organization of out-of-hours services

Definition: out-of-hours (OOH) is defined as 6.30pm–8.00am on weekdays, the whole weekend, Bank Holidays and public holidays. GPs have increasingly moved away from the traditional model of personally providing care 'around the clock'. There are several reasons for this:
- *Changed attitudes of GPs:* GPs find frequent on-call cover too onerous and an unacceptable intrusion into family life.
- *Daytime workload:* the role of the GP has shifted and ever more work comes the GP's way.
- *Number of OOH contacts:* today society has a '24-hour' culture. Consequently the number of GP OOH contacts has risen as has 'inappropriate' use of A&E services.

Since December 2004, PCOs have taken full responsibility for making sure there is effective OOH provision in the UK.

'Opting out' of OOH: both PMS and GMS practices can 'opt out' of providing an OOH service. The decision must be made for the whole practice—individual doctors within a practice cannot 'opt out' alone. The cost of opting out for a practice is 7% of the global sum (or PMS equivalent).

Provision of services during the OOH period by 'opted out' practices: there is nothing to stop practices that have opted out from offering surgeries or consultations within the time periods specified as OOH. These services can be paid for through the practice global sum or, by agreement with the PCO, may be paid for as an enhanced service.

Choice of OOH provider: PCOs can consider a range of alternative OOH care providers as long as accreditation standards are met. Only where a practice is exceptionally remote, can the PCO require a practice to continue providing OOH care. Special arrangements for payment then exist. *Several schemes operate side by side:*

In-practice rotas: traditional model of cover. Usually organized in a rota between practice GPs. Largely based on home visiting.

Extended rotas: GPs on-call in rotation for a small group of practices.

GP co-operatives: GPs grouped together (often >100 in a co-op) within a district to cover OOH care between themselves. In many cases run by local PCOs, and employing both GP principals and non-principals on a payment per session basis. Often several GPs are on call at any time— 1 doing visits; 1 taking calls; 1 seeing patients in a central clinic.

Hospital based OOH cover: GPs and primary care nurses in A&E departments.

Commercial OOH services: OOH provided by a commercial profit-making organization employing GPs and specialist nurses.

NHS Direct: 24 h, nurse-led telephone advice service available throughout the UK. It is designed as a first-line service and aims to have links to local primary care and OOH services. There is also an NHS Direct web site and advice booths in public places.

NHS Walk-in centres: walk-in clinics tend to offer nurse consultation and use NHS Direct algorithms. Most are sited in urban areas. They aim to provide easier access to medical care and are increasingly used to cover the OOH period.

Enhanced paramedic services: providing initial assessment of patients who are not able to get to OOH centres and/or patient transport to OOH centres.

Enhanced community nursing teams: providing care to patients who are terminally ill and initial assessment of patients who do not feel able to get to an OOH centre for other reasons.

The future of NHS OOH care: there is a move towards an integrated model of OOH care. One suggestion is that all OOH calls are routed through NHS Direct, which will act as a triage system—giving advice or directing callers to the appropriate service (e.g. A&E, ambulance call, GP OOH cover or routine GP appointment). The use of patient held 'smart cards' on which each patient's medical record could be stored will allow freer movement of patients between services without the danger of vital information being missed.

Further information

DoH The GMS Contract. ⊠ www.dh.gov.uk
NHS Direct. ☎ 0845 4647 ⊠ www.nhsdirect.nhs.uk
Separate services for Scotland and Wales can be accessed via this website.

Emergency patient encounters

Telephone consultations: the telephone is a useful way to answer simple queries without wasting valuable surgery time. Most GP surgeries now run telephone clinics, have telephone message books and/or bookable telephone slots in surgery time. Before giving advice, always ensure you have sufficient information upon which to base your judgement. If examination is needed, see the patient.

Emergency calls: nearly all requests for emergency care are made by telephone. *General rules:*

- *Train surgery staff* to handle distressed callers, recognize serious problems and act appropriately when such calls are received.
- *Where possible use a single number for patients to access help.* If using an answering machine ensure the message is easily heard and contains clear instructions. Worried patients find it difficult to cope with complicated telephone referral systems or messages.
- *Appear helpful* rather than defensive from the outset. Keep calm and friendly—even in the event of provocation. Worried callers often appear abrupt or demanding.
- *Record* the time of the call, date, patient's name, address and a contact telephone number, brief details of the problem, and action taken (even if calls are being recorded).
- *Collect only information you need to decide what action is necessary.* If the patient needs to be seen, collect enough information to decide where and how quickly the patient should be seen, and whether extra equipment or help is needed.
- *If giving advice*—make it simple and in language the patient can understand. Repeat to make sure it has been understood. Consider asking the patient/carer to repeat what you've told them. Always tell callers to ring back if symptoms change or they have further worries.
- *If a visit is indicated*—ensure the address is right and ask for directions if you are not sure where to go. Try to give a rough arrival time.
- *In some cases* (e.g. major trauma, large GI bleeds, MI, burns, overdoses) call for an emergency ambulance at once.
- *If a call seems inappropriate* consider the reason for it—e.g. depression might provoke recurrent calls for minor ailments.

⚠ If in doubt—see the patient.

Home visiting: home visits may be routine checks for housebound patients or emergency visits for patients temporarily unable to get to the surgery. Home visits done in working hours are usually done by practices under their GMS/PMS contract but in some areas home-visiting services are provided by the PCO and practices are able to 'opt out'.

Emergency visits

- Try to stick to the problem you've been called about.
- Take a concise history and examine as appropriate.
- Make a decision on management and explain it to the patient and any carers in clear and concise terms that they can understand. Repeat advice several times ± write it down.

- Record history, examination, management suggested, and advice given for the patient's notes.
- Always invite the patient and carers to ring you again should symptoms change, the situation deteriorate or further worries appear.
- For inappropriate calls, take time to educate the patient and/or carers about self-management and use of emergency GP visiting services.
- Always consider hidden reasons for seemingly unnecessary visits.

Being prepared
- Ensure you have a reliable car with a full tank of fuel
- Have a good street map of the area ± Ordinance Survey map
- Carry a large, strong torch in the car and a mobile telephone
- Check your drug box is fully stocked and all items are in date, and that all equipment carried is operational; carry spare batteries
- Carry a list of emergency telephone numbers
- Know which chemists have extended opening hours and/or carry the chemist's rota.

Safety and security
- In all cases ensure someone else knows where you are going, when to expect you back and what to do if you don't return on time.
- If going to a call you are worried about either take someone with you to sit in the car or call the police to meet you there before going in.
- If you reach a call and find you are uncomfortable, make sure you can get out. Note the layout of the property and make sure you have a clear route to the door.
- Set up your mobile phone to call the police or your base at a single touch of a button. Consider carrying an attack alarm.
- If possible have separate bags for drugs and consultation equipment.
- Leave the drug box locked out of sight in the boot of the car when doing a visit.

Referral letters: good communication is essential when referring patients to other doctors and agencies. Ensure all referral letters include:
- Address of the referrer (including telephone number if possible)
- Name and address of registered GP if not the referrer
- Date of referral
- Name, address and date of birth of the patient (and any other identifiers available, e.g. hospital or NHS number)
- Name of the person to whom the patient is being referred (or department if not a named individual)
- Presenting condition—history, examination, investigations already performed with results, treatments already tried with outcomes.
- Relevant past medical history and family history
- Current medication and any intolerances/allergies known
- Reason for referral (what you want the recipient of the letter to do), e.g. to investigate symptoms, to reassure parents
- Any other relevant information, e.g. social circumstances
- Signature (and name in legible format) of referrer.

❶ Consider using carbonized paper to keep copies of referral letters.

Equipment and drugs

Resuscitation equipment and drugs: see Table 1.1
- Resuscitation equipment is used relatively infrequently. Staff must know where to find equipment and be trained to use the equipment to a level appropriate to the individual's expected role.
- Each practice should have a named individual with responsibility for checking the state of readiness of all resuscitation drugs and equipment, on a regular basis, ideally once a week. In common with drugs, disposable items like the adhesive electrodes have a finite shelf life and will require replacement from time to time if unused.

The doctor's bag: consider including the following (exact contents will vary according to location and circumstances):

Diagnostic equipment
- Stethoscope
- Sphygmomanometer
- Thermometer
- Gloves, jelly and tissues
- Torch
- Otoscope
- Ophthalmoscope
- Tongue depressors
- Peak flow meter
- Pulse oximeter
- Fluorescein sticks
- Urine and blood dipsticks
- Tourniquet, vacutainer (or syringe) and needles
- Patella hammer
- Swabs
- Specimen containers
- Vaginal speculum ± sponge forceps
- Foetal stethoscope/Doppler.

Administrative equipment
- Mobile telephone ± charger
- Controlled drugs record book
- Envelopes
- Headed notepaper
- Local map
- Pathology/X-ray forms
- Prescription pad
- List of useful telephone numbers
- BNF/Mimms
- Quick reference text, e.g. *Oxford Handbook of General Practice*
- Obstetric calculator
- Peak flow chart/wheel
- Book/cards/adhesive strips/carbonized paper for keeping a record of patient encounters
- Temporary resident records
- List of local chemists and out of hours opening times
- Small amount of change for public telephones, parking, etc.

Other equipment
- Airway ± Laerdal mask
- Oxygen cylinder and mask with reservoir bag
- Automated external defibrillator
- Nebulizer
- Spacer device
- IV cannula
- IV giving set and fluids
- Needles/syringes
- Bandages
- Gauze swabs
- Adhesive plasters
- Scissors
- Steristrips
- Suturing equipment/skin glue
- Urinary catheter and bag
- Antiseptic sachets
- Dressing pack
- Sharps box.

Table 1.1 Resuscitation equipment needed

Equipment	Notes
Defibrillator with electrodes and razor	An automated external defibrillator should be available wherever and whenever sick patients are seen
	Regular maintenance is needed even if the machine is not used
	After the machine is used the manufacturers' instructions should be followed to return it to a state of readiness with minimum delay
Pocket mask with 1-way valve	All personnel should be trained to use one
Oro-pharyngeal airway	Suitable for use by those appropriately trained. Keep a range of sizes available
Oxygen and mask with reservoir bag	Should be available wherever possible ⚠ If carrying oxygen in your car, the car must be marked with appropriate symbols in case of accident, and you must inform your insurance company
	Oxygen cylinders need regular maintenance—follow national safety standards
Suction	Simple, mechanical, portable, hand-held suction devices are recommended
Drugs	Epinephrine/adrenaline—1 mg IV
	Atropine—3 mg IV (give once only)—for bradycardia, asystole and pulseless electrical activity
	Amiodarone—300 mg IV—for VF resistant to defibrillation
	Naloxone—for suspected cases of respiratory arrest due to opiate overdose
	⚠ There is no evidence for the use of alkalizing agents, buffers or calcium salts before hospitalization
	Drugs should be given by the IV route, preferably through a catheter placed in a large vein, for example in the antecubital fossa, and flushed in with a bolus of IV fluid
	Many drugs may be given via the bronchial route if a tracheal tube is in place; for epinephrine/adrenaline and atropine the dose is double the IV dose
Other	Saline flush, gloves, syringes and needles, IV cannulae, IV fluids, sharps box, scissors, tape

❶ Practices are rewarded with quality points for inspection, calibration, maintenance and replacement of equipment (Management Indicator 7) and for having a system for checking the expiry dates of emergency drugs (Medicines Indicator 3).

Drugs for the doctor's bag: the GP's bag must be lockable and not left unattended during home visits. If left in the car keep the bag locked and out of sight—preferably in the boot. Consider having a separate bag for drugs and consultation equipment and only get the drug bag out of the boot of the car if it is needed. Keep the bag away from extremes of temperature. *Consider:*

Injectables
- Adrenaline (epinephrine)
- Atropine
- Amiodarone
- Benzylpenicillin injection
- Cefotaxime injection
- Lorazepam/diazepam
- NSAID, e.g. diclofenac
- Local anaesthetic, e.g. lidocaine
- Opioid analgesic, e.g. morphine, pethidine, diamorphine
- Naloxone
- Antiemetic, e.g. domperidone, prochlorperazine
- Antihistamine, e.g. chlorphenamine
- Hydrocortisone injection
- Diuretic, e.g. furosemide
- Syntometrine
- Glucagon ± IV glucose
- Major tranquillizer, e.g. haloperidol, chlorpromazine
- Thrombolytic therapy (if >½ h from nearest acute hospital and have training)

Oral drugs
- Antacid
- Antibiotics (adult tablets and paediatric sachets), e.g. amoxicillin + erythromycin/clarithromycin
- Antihistamine
- Rehydration tablets/sachets
- Aspirin
- Lorazepam
- Paracetamol tablets + suspension
- Prednisolone tablets (soluble)
- NSAID, e.g. ibuprofen

Other drugs
- GTN spray
- Bronchodilator for nebulizer
- Salbutamol inhaler + spacer
- Antibiotic eye drops
- Hypostop glucose gel
- Glycerol suppositories
- Rectal diazepam
- Diclofenac suppositories
- Domperidone suppositories

⚠ Check drugs at least 2×/y to see they are still in date and usable. Record origin, batch number and expiry date of *all* drugs administered to patients or dispensed to them to take themselves.

Further information

Drugs & Therapeutics Bulletin Drugs for the doctor's bag 1—Adults (September 2005) and Drugs for the doctor's bag 2—Children (November 2005) www.dtb.bmj.com

Drugs given to patients from the doctor's bag should be in a suitable container and properly labelled with:

- Patient's name
- Drug name
- Drug dosage
- Quantity of tablets
- Instructions on use
- Relevant warnings
- Name and address of the doctor
- Date
- Warning 'Keep out of reach of children'

Resuscitation

Managing a resuscitation attempt outside hospital

⚠ **Importance of resuscitation training**

- Ventricular fibrillation complicating acute MI is the most common cause of cardiac arrest that members of the primary health care team will encounter.
- Success is greatest when the event is witnessed and attempted defibrillation is performed with the minimum of delay.
- It is unacceptable for patients who sustain a cardiopulmonary arrest on a GP premises to await the arrival of the ambulance service before basic resuscitation is performed and a defibrillator is available.

❶ Practices can claim quality points for training practice employed clinical staff (Education Indicator 1) and non-clinical staff (Education Indicator 5) in basic life support skills.

Automated external defibrillators (AEDs)

- Modern AEDs have simplified the process of defibrillation considerably.
- The use of such machines should be within the capabilities of all medical and nursing staff working in the community so ALL practices should have an AED.
- Increasingly, trained lay persons are successfully employing AEDs and it is quite appropriate for reception, administrative and secretarial staff to be trained in their use.

Ethical issues

- It is essential to identify individuals in whom cardiopulmonary arrest is a terminal event and where resuscitation is inappropriate.
- Overall responsibility for a 'Do not attempt to resuscitate (DNAR)' decision rests with the doctor in charge of the patient's care.
- Seek opinions of other members of the medical and nursing team, the patient and any relatives in reaching a DNAR decision.
- Record the patient should not be resuscitated in the notes, the reasons for that decision and what the relatives have been told.
- Ensure all members of the multidisciplinary team involved with the patient's care are aware of the decision and record it in their notes.
- Review the decision not to attempt resuscitation regularly in the light of the patient's condition.

Essential reading

BMA, RCN and Resuscitation Council (UK) Decisions relating to cardio-pulmonary resuscitation (2001) ⌨ www.resus.org.uk

⊛ Basic adult life support

Basic paediatric life support: 📖 p.24.

Basic adult life support (BLS): is a holding operation—sustaining life until help arrives. BLS should be started as soon as the arrest is detected—outcome is less good the longer the delay.

1. **Danger:** ensure safety of rescuer and patient.

2. **Response:** check the patient for any response
• Is he **A**lert? Yes/No
• Does he respond to **V**ocal stimuli? Yes/No
• Does he respond to a **P**ainful stimulus (pinching the lower part of the nasal septum)? Yes/No
• Is the patient **U**nconscious? Yes/No

If he responds by answering or moving: don't move the patient unless in danger. Get help. Reassess regularly.

If he does not respond: shout for help; turn the patient onto his back.

3. **Airways:** open the airways—place one hand on the patient's forehead and tilt his head back. With fingertips under the point of the patient's chin, lift the chin to open the airways.

⚠ Try to avoid head tilt if trauma to the neck is suspected

4. **Breathing:** with airways open, look, listen and feel for breathing for no more than 10 sec—look for chest movement, listen at the victim's mouth for breath sounds, feel for air on your cheek.

If breathing normally: turn the patient into the recovery position (📖 p.30), get help and check for continued breathing.

If not breathing or only making occasional gasps/weak attempts at breathing: get help then start chest compressions.

❶ In the first few minutes after cardiac arrest, a victim may be barely breathing, or taking infrequent, noisy, gasps. Don't confuse this with normal breathing. If you have any doubt whether breathing is normal, act as if it is *not* normal.

5. **Circulation:** start chest compressions if not breathing:
• Kneel by the side of the victim and place the heel of 1 hand in the centre of the victim's chest. Place the heel of your other hand on top of the first hand. Interlock the fingers of your hands and ensure that pressure is not applied over the victim's ribs. Don't apply any pressure over the upper abdomen or the bottom end of the bony sternum.
• Position yourself vertically above the victim's chest and, with arms straight, press down on the sternum 4–5 cm.
• After each compression, release all the pressure on the chest without losing contact between your hands and the sternum. Compression and release should take an equal amount of time
• Repeat at a rate of ~100×/min.

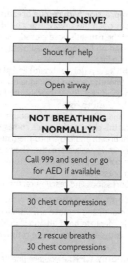

Fig. 2.1 Adult basic life support (ABLS) algorithm.

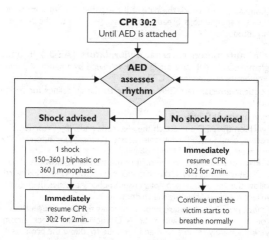

Fig. 2.2 Automated external defibrillator (AED) algorithm.

Figures 2.1 and 2.2 are reproduced from the Resuscitation guidelines (2005) with permission
🖳 www.resus.org.uk

6. **Combine chest compression with rescue breaths:**
- After 30 compressions open the airways using head tilt and chin lift.
- Pinch the soft part of the patient's nose closed, using the index finger and thumb of your hand on his forehead. Allow the patient's mouth to open, but maintain chin lift.
- Give a rescue breath—take a normal breath and place your lips around the patient's mouth (mouth-to-nose technique is an alternative) making sure that you have a good seal. Blow steadily into his mouth for ~1 sec while watching for the chest to rise.
- Maintaining head tilt and chin lift, take your mouth away from the patient and watch for the chest to fall as air comes out.
- Take another normal breath and blow into the patient's mouth again to give a total of 2 effective rescue breaths. Then return your hands without delay to the correct position on the sternum and give a further 30 chest compressions.
- Continue chest compressions and rescue breaths in a ratio of 30:2.

If rescue breaths don't make the chest rise:
- Check the patient's mouth and remove any visible obstruction.
- Recheck that there is adequate head tilt and chin lift.
- Don't attempt >2 breaths each time before returning to chest compressions.

Chest-compression-only CPR: if you are unable or unwilling to give rescue breaths, give continuous chest compressions only, at a rate of 100/min.

⚠ Only stop to recheck the patient if the patient makes a movement or takes a spontaneous breath; otherwise resuscitation should not be interrupted

Use of automated external defibrillators (AEDs) in adults: program AEDs to deliver a single shock followed by a pause of 2 min for the immediate resumption of CPR.

If a patient arrests: start CPR according to the guidelines for basic life support.

As soon as the AED arrives:
- Switch on the AED and attach the electrode pads. If >1 rescuer is present, continue CPR while this is done. (Some AEDs automatically switch on when the AED lid is opened).
  - Place one AED pad to the right of the sternum, below the clavicle.
  - Place the other pad in the mid-axillary line with its long axis vertical
- Follow the voice/visual prompts. Ensure nobody touches the victim while the AED is analysing the rhythm.

If a shock is indicated: ensure nobody touches the victim. Push the shock button as directed (fully-automatic AEDs deliver the shock automatically). Immediately resume CPR and continue to follow the prompts.

If no shock is indicated: immediately resume CPR and continue to follow the prompts.

Use of AEDs in children: 📖 p.26

When to go for assistance: it is vital for rescuers to get assistance as quickly as possible. If you are the only rescuer, go for assistance before starting CPR.

When >1 rescuer is available
- One should start resuscitation while another goes for assistance
- Another should take over CPR every 2 min to prevent fatigue. Ensure minimum of delay during changeover of rescuers.

Duration of resuscitation: continue resuscitation until:
- Qualified help arrives and takes over
- The victim starts breathing normally *and/or*
- You become exhausted.

Pad position for external defibrillators: place 1 pad to the right of the sternum below the clavicle. Place the other pad vertically in the mid-axillary line approximately level with the V6 ECG electrode position or female breast (though clear of any breast tissue)

Further reading

Resuscitation Council (UK) Resuscitation guidelines (2005) 🖥 www.resus.org.uk

☼: **Advanced adult life support**

Advanced life support has 3 basic stages:
- Revive the patient using basic life support (📖 p.18). Basic life support should be started if there is any delay in obtaining a defibrillator, but must not delay shock delivery.
- Restore spontaneous cardiac output, using an automatic external defibrillator (📖 p.20) or manual defibrillator.
- Review possible causes for cardiac arrest and take further action as needed.

Precordial thump: appropriate if the arrest is witnessed and a defibrillator is not to hand—may dislodge a pulmonary embolus or 'jerk' the heart back into sinus rhythm. Use the ulnar edge of a tightly clenched fist and deliver a sharp impact to the lower ½ of the sternum from a height of ~20 cm then immediately retract the fist.

VF/VT arrest
- Attempt defibrillation (1 shock 150–200 J biphasic or 360 J monophasic).
- Immediately resume chest compressions (30:2) without reassessing rhythm or feeling for the pulse. Continue CPR for 2 min then pause briefly to check the monitor.
- If VT/VF persists give a 2nd shock (150–360 J biphasic or 360 J monophasic), continue CPR for 2 min then pause briefly to check the monitor.
- If VT/VF persists give adrenaline (epinephrine) 1 mg IV (or intraosseously if IV access cannot be attained) followed immediately by a 3rd shock (150–360 J biphasic or 360 J monophasic). Resume CPR immediately and continue for 2 min then pause briefly to check the monitor.
- If VF/VT persists give amiodarone 300 mg IV (lidocaine 1 mg/kg is an alternative if amiodarone isn't available) followed immediately by a 4th shock (150–360 J biphasic or 360 J monophasic). Resume CPR immediately and continue for 2 min.
- Give adrenaline (epinephrine) 1 mg IV immediately before alternate shocks (i.e. approximately every 3–5 min).
- Give a further shock after each 2 min period of CPR and after confirming that VF/VT persists.

Non-VT/VF arrest
- Start CPR 30:2. Without stopping CPR, check that the leads are attached correctly.
- Give adrenaline (epinephrine) 1 mg IV as soon as IV access is achieved.
- If asystole or pulseless electrical activity with rate <60 beats/min, give atropine 3 mg IV (once only).
- Continue CPR 30:2 until the airways is secured, then continue chest compression without pausing during ventilation.
- Recheck the rhythm after 2 min and proceed accordingly.
- Give adrenaline (epinephrine) 1 mg IV every 3–5 min (alternate loops).

Fine VF: fine VF difficult to distinguish from asystole is very unlikely to be shocked successfully into a perfusing rhythm. Continuing good quality CPR may improve the amplitude and frequency of the VF and improve the chance of successful defibrillation to a perfusing rhythm.

Organized electrical activity: if organized electrical activity is seen during the brief pause in compressions, check for a pulse.
• If a pulse is present, start post-resuscitation care (📖 p.30).
• If no pulse, continue CPR and follow the non-shockable algorithm.

Further reading
Resuscitation Council (UK) Resuscitation guidelines (2005) 🖳 www.resus.org.uk

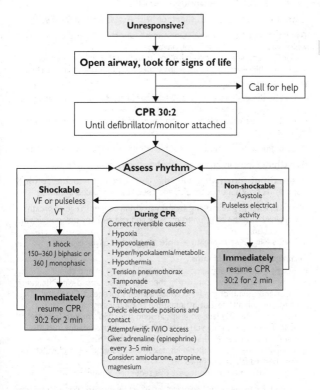

Fig. 2.3 Adult advanced life support algorithm.

Figures 2.3–2.5 are reproduced from Resuscitation guidelines (2005) with permission. Full version available from 🖳 www.resus.org.uk

:☼: **Basic paediatric life support**

Basic paediatric life support is a holding operation until help arrives.

Danger: ensure safety of rescuer and patient

Response: check the child for any response
- Is he **A**lert?
- Does he respond to **V**ocal stimuli?
- Does he respond to **P**ainful stimuli (pinch lower part of nasal septum)?
- Is he **U**nconscious?

If he responds by answering or moving: don't move the child unless in danger. Get help. Reassess regularly.

If he does not respond: shout for help. Assess airways (below)

Airways: open the airways. Don't move the child from the position in which you found him unless you have to.
- Gently tilt the head back—with your hand on the child's forehead
- Lift the chin—with your fingertips under the point of the child's chin.

If unsuccessful:
- Try jaw thrust—place the first 2 fingers of each hand behind each side of the child's jaw bone and push the jaw forward.
- Try lifting the chin or jaw thrust after carefully turning the child on to his back.

⚠ Avoid head tilt as much as possible if trauma to the neck is suspected

Breathing: look, listen and feel for breathing (maximum 10 sec)

If breathing normally: turn the child carefully into the recovery position (📖 p.30) if unconscious, and check for continued breathing

If not breathing or making agonal gasps (infrequent irregular breaths):
- Carefully turn the child on to his back and remove any obvious airway obstruction.
- Give 5 initial rescue breaths—note any gag or cough response.

Technique for rescue breaths:
- Ensure head tilt (neutral position for children <1 y) and chin lift.
- If age ≥1 y, pinch the soft part of the child's nose closed with the index finger and thumb of the hand which is on his forehead. Open the child's mouth a little, but maintain the chin upwards.
- Take a breath and place your lips around the child's mouth (mouth and nose if <1 y[1]), ensuring you have a good seal. Blow steadily into the child's airway over ~1–1.5 sec watching for chest rise.
- Maintaining head tilt and chin lift, take your mouth away and watch for the chest to fall as air comes out.
- Take another breath and repeat this sequence 5 times.

❶ If you have difficulty achieving an effective breath, consider airway obstruction—📖 p.74

---

1 If the nose and mouth can't both be covered, place your lips around the mouth alone as for an older child, or nose alone (close the child's lips to prevent air escape).

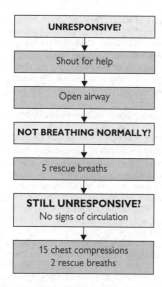

After 1 minute call for help then continue CPR

Fig. 2.4 Paediatric basic life support (PBLS) algorithm.

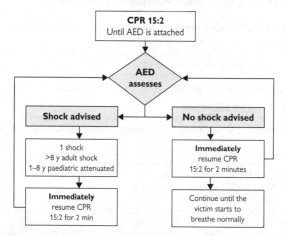

Fig. 2.5 Automated external defibrillator (AED) algorithm.

Circulation (signs of life): check (maximum 10 sec) for:
- Any movement, coughing or normal breathing (not agonal gasps)
- Pulse—child ≥1 y carotid pulse; child <1 y brachial pulse.

If circulation is present: continue rescue breathing until the child starts breathing effectively on his own. Turn the child into the recovery position (📖 p.30) if unconscious, and reassess frequently.

If circulation is absent: or slow pulse (<60 beats/min) with poor perfusion, or you are not sure:
- Give 15 chest compressions. Then give 2 rescue breaths followed by 15 further chest compressions.
- Continue the cycle of 2 breaths followed by 15 chest compressions.

❶ Lone rescuers may use a ratio of 30 compressions:2 rescue breaths

Technique for chest compressions: compress the sternum 1 finger's breadth above the xiphisternum by ~$^1/_3$ of the depth of the chest. Release the pressure then repeat at a rate of ~100 compressions/min.
- Children <1 y with a lone rescuer: use the tips of 2 fingers
- Children <1 y with ≥2 rescuers: place both thumbs flat on the lower $^1/_3$ of the sternum with tips pointing towards the child's head and encircle the lower part of the child's ribcage with the tips of the fingers supporting the infant's back. Press down with both thumbs.
- Children >1 y: place the heel of 1 hand over the lower $^1/_3$ of the sternum. Lift the fingers. Position yourself vertically above the chest with arm straight, and push downwards. For larger children use both hands with fingers interlocked to achieve satisfactory compressions.

⚠ Stop to recheck for signs of a circulation only if the child moves or takes a spontaneous breath—otherwise continue uninterrupted

Use of automated external defibrillators (AEDs) in children
- Children >8 y: use the standard adult AED.
- Children aged 1–8 y: paediatric pads or a paediatric mode should be used if available—if not, use the adult AED as it is.
- Children <1 y: AED use is currently not advised.

If a patient arrests: start CPR according to the guidelines for PBLS.

As soon as the AED arrives:
- Switch on the AED and attach the electrode pads. If >1 rescuer is present, continue CPR while this is done. (Some AEDs automatically switch on when the AED lid is opened.)
  - Place one AED pad to the right of the sternum, below the clavicle.
  - Place the other pad in the mid-axillary line with its long axis vertical
- Follow the voice/visual prompts. Ensure nobody touches the victim while the AED is analysing the rhythm.

If a shock is indicated: ensure nobody touches the victim. Push the shock button as directed (fully-automatic AEDs deliver the shock automatically). Immediately resume CPR and continue to follow the prompts.
If no shock is indicated: immediately resume CPR and continue to follow the prompts.

When to go for assistance: it is vital for rescuers to get assistance as quickly as possible when a child collapses.

When >1 rescuer is available: one should start resuscitation while another rescuer goes for assistance.

Lone rescuer: perform resuscitation for 1 min before going for assistance (and consider taking a young child/infant with you to minimize interruption in CPR). The only exception to this is a witnessed sudden collapse—as in this case cardiac arrest is likely to be due to arrhythmia and the child may need defibrillation so seek help immediately.

Duration of resuscitation: continue resuscitation until:
- child shows signs of life (spontaneous respiration, pulse, movement)
- further qualified help arrives
- you become exhausted

Cervical spine injury
- If spinal cord injury is suspected (e.g. if the victim has sustained a fall, been struck on the head or neck, or has been rescued after diving into shallow water) take particular care during handling and resuscitation to maintain alignment of the head, neck and chest in the neutral position.
- A spinal board and/or cervical collar should be used if available.

Resuscitation of the newborn: 📖 p.200.

Further information
Resuscitation Council (UK) Resuscitation guidelines (2005) 🖥 www.resus.org.uk

☼ Advanced paediatric life support

Cardiac arrest in children is rare. Unless there is underlying heart disease, it is usually a consequence of respiratory arrest, which results in asystole or pulseless electrical activity and has poor prognosis. Good airway management and providing high flow oxygen for very sick children is therefore important in preventing cardiac arrest.

Basic paediatric life support: follow the algorithm on ☐ p.25.

Unable to ventilate? Consider foreign body in the airway and initiate airway obstruction sequence—☐ p.74.

Checking the pulse

- Child—feel for the carotid pulse in the neck.
- Infant—feel for the brachial pulse on the inner aspect of the upper arm.

Once the airway is protected: if the airway is protected by tracheal intubation, continue chest compression without pausing for ventilation. Provide ventilation at a rate of 10/min and compression at 100/min. When circulation is restored, ventilate the child at a rate of 12–20 breaths/min.

Adrenaline (epinephrine) dose

- IV or interosseous (IO) access—10 mcgm/kg adrenaline (0.1 ml/kg of 1:10 000 solution).
- If circulatory access is not present, and can't be quickly obtained, but the child has a tracheal tube in place, consider giving adrenaline 100 mcgm/kg via the tracheal tube (1 ml/kg of 1:10 000 or 0.1 ml/kg of 1:1000 solution). This is the least satisfactory route of administration.

⚠ Don't give 1:1000 adrenaline IV or IO.

VF/Pulseless VT: less common in paediatric life support.
- Defibrillation:
  - Give 1 shock of 4 J/kg or
  - If using an AED for a child of 1–8 y deliver a paediatric attenuated adult shock energy.
  - If using an AED for a child >8 y use the adult shock energy.
- For VF/pulseless VT persisting after the 3rd shock, try amiodarone 5 mg/kg diluted in 5% dextrose.

Bradycardia: when bradycardia is unresponsive to improved ventilation and circulatory support, try atropine 20 mcgm/kg (maximum dose 600 mcgm; minimum dose 100 mcgm).

Magnesium: magnesium treatment is indicated in children with documented hypomagnesaemia or with polymorphic VT ('torsade de pointes'), regardless of cause. Give IV magnesium sulphate over several minutes at a dose of 25–50 mg/kg (to a maximum of 2 g).

Intravenous fluids: in situations where the cardiac arrest has resulted from circulatory failure, a standard (20 ml/kg) bolus of crystalloid fluid should be given if there is no response to the initial dose of epinephrine.

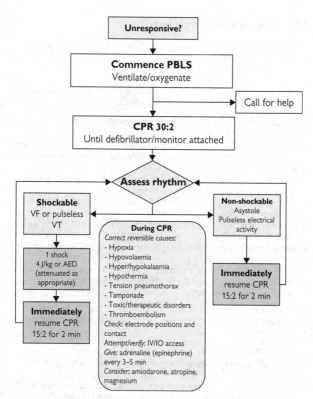

Fig. 2.6 Paediatric advanced life support (PALS) algorithm.

Estimating the weight of a child for drug/fluid doses

- May not be necessary—use a recent weight from the parent-held child record if available.
- Otherwise for children >1 y, weight (in kg) ≈2× (age +4).

:Ö: **Recovery position**

When circulation and breathing have been restored, it is important to:
- Maintain a good airway
- Ensure the tongue does not cause obstruction
- Minimize the risk of inhalation of gastric contents.

For this reason the victim should be placed in the recovery position. This allows the tongue to fall forward, keeping the airway clear.

Putting a patient in the recovery position: see Figure 2.7
- Remove the patient's glasses
- Kneel beside the patient and make sure that both legs are straight (A)
- Place the arm nearest to you out at right angles to the body, elbow bent with the hand palm uppermost (A)
- Bring the far arm across the chest, and hold the back of the hand against the patient's cheek nearest to you (B)
- With your other hand, grasp the far leg just above the knee and pull it up, keeping the foot on the ground (B)
- Keeping the patient's hand pressed against his cheek, pull on the leg to roll the patient towards you on to his side (C)
- Adjust the upper leg so that both the hip and knee are bent at right angles (D)
- Tilt the head back to make sure the airway remain open (D)
- Adjust the hand under the cheek, if necessary, to keep the head tilted
- Check breathing regularly.

⚠ Monitor the peripheral circulation of the lower arm. If the patient has to be kept in the recovery position for >30 min, turn the patient on to the opposite side.

The unconscious child
- The child should be in as near a true lateral position as possible with his mouth dependant to allow free drainage of fluid
- The position should be stable. In an infant this may require the support of a small pillow or rolled up blanket placed behind the infant's back to maintain the position.

Cervical spine injury
- If spinal cord injury is suspected (e.g. if the victim has sustained a fall, been struck on the head or neck, or has been rescued after diving into shallow water) take particular care during handling and resuscitation to maintain alignment of the head, neck and chest in the neutral position.
- A spinal board and/or cervical collar should be used if available.

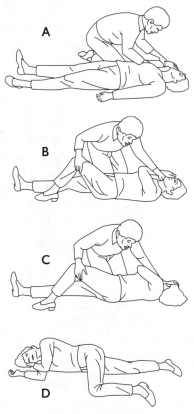

Fig. 2.7 The recovery position.

Figure 2.7 is reproduced with permission from Stoke-on-Trent drugs and alcohol action team.

Other acute emergencies

:☼: Road Traffic Accidents (RTAs) and other major traumatic incidents

Doctors are not legally obliged to attend an accident they happen to pass—but most feel morally obliged to do so.

Immediate action
- Assess the scene.
- Ensure police and ambulance have been called.
- Take steps to ensure your own safety and that of others, e.g. park your vehicle defensively; turn on hazard lights; use warning triangles.
- Ensure all vehicle ignitions are turned off.
- Triage casualties into priority groups—decide who to attend first.
- Forbid smoking.

Immediate treatment
- Check the need for basic resuscitation:
  - Airways patent?
  - Breathing adequate?
  - Circulation intact?
- Resuscitate as necessary (📖 p.18–31 or inside back cover).
- Control any haemorrhage with elevation and pressure.
- DO NOT attempt to move anyone who potentially could have a back or neck injury until skilled personnel and equipment are available.
- Do not give anything by mouth.
- Use coats and rugs to keep victims warm.
- If available give analgesia (e.g. opioids—but not if significant head injury or risk of intraperitoneal injury; entonox—from ambulance).
- If shocked, set up IV fluids if available.
- Take directions from the paramedics—they are almost certainly more experienced than you in these situations.

Medicolegal issues
- Ensure your medicolegal insurance covers emergency treatments.
- Keep full records of events, action taken, drugs administered, origin of drugs, batch numbers and expiry dates.
- A GP can charge a fee to the victims for any assistance given.

Burns and scalds: 📖 p.230.

Drowning: 📖 p.233.

Head injury: 📖 p.222.

Fractures: 📖 p.219.

Post-traumatic stress disorder (PTSD): caused by experiencing or witnessing a traumatic event, e.g. major accident, fire, assault, military combat. It is estimated 25–30% of those witnessing such events go on to develop PTSD. It can affect people of all ages.

Symptoms: most develop symptoms immediately after the event though onset of symptoms can be delayed (<15%). However, it is common for sufferers not to present until months or years after onset of symptoms despite the considerable distress caused by them. Symptoms may be misdiagnosed as depression or anxiety. *4 main symptom clusters:*

- *Intrusive recollections*—thoughts; nightmares; flashbacks
- *Avoidant behaviour*—avoidance of people, places, situations or circumstances resembling or associated with the event; refusal to talk or think about the event; excessive rumination about questions that prevent them coming to terms with the event (e.g. Why me? How could it have been prevented?)
- *Hyperarousal*—↑ anxiety and irritability, insomnia, poor concentration, hypervigilance.
- *Numbing of emotions*—lack of ability to experience feelings; feeling detached from other people; giving up previously significant activities; amnesia for significant parts of the event.

Nearly $^2/_3$ experience chronic symptoms and there is a strong association with other psychiatric conditions especially depression, anxiety and drug/alcohol abuse and dependence.

Management: treat any other associated psychiatric illness.

- *Watchful waiting:* appropriate for patients with mild symptoms that have been present for <4 wk after the trauma. Be supportive and listen. Arrange a follow-up contact within 1 mo.
- *Trauma-focused psychological treatment* (trauma focused cognitive behavioural therapy and/or eye movement desensitization and reprocessing (EMDR): refer (usually via the community mental health team) all patients with severe symptoms <4 wk after the trauma or if ongoing symptoms beyond 4 wk that affect every day life.
- *Drug treatment:* should not be used as a routine first-line treatment in preference to a trauma-focused psychological therapy. Reserve for those with continuing symptoms despite trauma-focused psychological therapy or who have refused trauma-focused psychological therapy. Drug treatments include paroxetine, mirtazapine (unlicensed), amitriptyline (consultant initiation only—unlicensed) and phenelzine (consultant initiation only—unlicensed).

❶ Debriefing immediately after the traumatic event is unhelpful. NICE recommends screening using screening questionnaires for those at particularly high risk of developing PTSD, e.g. those involved in a major disaster or refugees. In those cases, screening should be organized by the relevant authorities, e.g. those responsible for the local disaster plan or refugee centres.

Further reading

NICE Post-traumatic stress disorder (PTSD): the management of PTSD in adults and children in primary, secondary and community care (2005) ⬚ www.nice.org.uk

⊛ Acute pain in emergency situations

Assessment of pain: take a history to ascertain:
- what the patient means when s/he complains of pain
- the cause of the pain
- the severity of the pain.

❶ Don't jump to conclusions or make assumptions about a patient's pain. To make an accurate assessment listen carefully to the history—even if the clinical scenario is one you've encountered numerous times before, or the patient is one you have met many times before.

Assessment questions: there are many approaches to assessing pain. The specifics of each scheme are not crucial—but it is important the scheme used has a logical outline that works for the individual clinician. A simple mnemonic approach is detailed opposite (Figure 3.1).

Elderly patients and patients with difficulty communicating: high prevalence of pain in the elderly population is now well recognized. 40–80% of elderly people in institutions are in pain. The reason for this lies in the difficulty in assessing those with communication difficulties. Additionally, the elderly often minimize their pain making it even more difficult to evaluate.

Methods of evaluation: unusual behaviour and its return to normal with adequate analgesia may be the only confirmation of pain in patients with communication difficulties. Examples include:

Verbal expression, e.g.
- crying when touched
- shouting
- becoming very quiet
- swearing
- grunting
- talking without making sense

Facial expression, e.g.
- grimacing/wincing
- closing eyes
- worried expression
- withdrawn/no expression

Behavioural expression, e.g.
- jumping on touch
- hand pointing to body area
- increasing confusion
- rocking/shaking
- not eating
- staying in bed/chair
- grumpy mood

Physical expression, e.g.
- cold
- pale
- clammy
- change in colour
- change in vital signs if acute pain (e.g. BP, pulse)

Examine the patient: the cause of the problem may be clear to you from history alone but examine the patient to confirm/refute your proposed diagnosis.

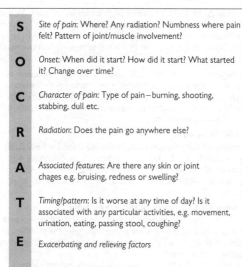

S — *Site of pain*: Where? Any radiation? Numbness where pain felt? Pattern of joint/muscle involvement?

O — *Onset*: When did it start? How did it start? What started it? Change over time?

C — *Character of pain*: Type of pain – burning, shooting, stabbing, dull etc.

R — *Radiation*: Does the pain go anywhere else?

A — *Associated features*: Are there any skin or joint chages e.g. bruising, redness or swelling?

T — *Timing/pattern*: Is it worse at any time of day? Is it associated with any particular activities, e.g. movement, urination, eating, passing stool, coughing?

E — *Exacerbating and relieving factors*

S — *Severity*: Record especially if the pain is chronic and you want to measure change over time, consider a patient diary. Ask about:
- Pain intensity e.g. none-mild-moderate-severe; rank on a 1–10 scale.
- Record interference with sleep or usual activities.
- Pain relief e.g. none-slight-moderate-good-complete.

Fig. 3.1 Points to consider when taking a history of pain.

Pain assessment tools: sometimes it is helpful to use pain scales to assess the degree of pain that a patient is in—particularly if communication is difficult. Figure 3.2 is a simple visual analogue pain scale—ask patients to point to the place on the line that represents how much pain they are in. 10 is the most possible pain and 0, no pain.

The analgesic ladder: treat the cause of the pain wherever possible. If the cause of the pain is untreatable or treatable in the community, most pain can be managed using a step-by-step approach (Figure 3.3, 📖 p.41). Start at the step that corresponds to the current pain level and step up or down as necessary.

Step 1: mild pain—non-opioid
- Start treatment with paracetamol. Stress the need for REGULAR dosage. Adult dose is 1 g every 4–6 h (maximum daily dose 4 g).
- If this is not adequate, either try a NSAID, e.g. ibuprofen 400 mg tds (if appropriate) alone or in combination with paracetamol, or proceed to step 2.

Step 2: moderate pain—weak opioid ± non-opioid
- Start treatment with a combined preparation of paracetamol with codeine or dihydrocodeine. Combining 2 analgesics with different mechanisms of action enables better pain control than using either drug alone at that dose.
- Combinations have ↓ dose-related side-effects but the range of side-effects is ↑ (additive effects of 2 drugs).
- Combinations using 30 mg of codeine (e.g. solpadol) are more effective than paracetamol alone but it is cheaper and more flexible if constituents are prescribed separately, e.g. 'paracetamol 500 mg/codeine 30 mg'.
- Consider a NSAID in addition if pain is inflammatory or musculoskeletal and no contraindications.
- Advise patients to take tablets regularly and not to assess efficacy after only a couple of doses.

❶ There is no proven additional analgesic benefit using paracetamol + 8 mg of codeine, compared with paracetamol alone.

Step 3: Strong opioid ± non-opioid
- *For acute severe pain:* consider use of an IM/IV/s/cut/PR opioid, e.g. diamorphine 5 mg (10 mg for heavier patients) s/cut or IM or morphine 10 mg (15 mg for heavier patients) s/cut or IM. If the patient is shocked or has peripheral vasoconstriction, diamorphine can be given by slow IV injection (1.25–5 mg at a rate of 1 mg/min) as can morphine (2.5–7.5 mg at a rate of 2 mg/min).
- *For more chronic severe pain:* use immediate release morphine tablets or morphine solution po. 2 tablets of co-codamol contain 60 mg of codeine, which is equi-analgesic to ~6 mg of oral morphine. If changing to morphine, use a minimum dose of 5 mg (6 mg is hard to prescribe). ↑ the dose upwards by 30–50% every 24 h until pain is controlled or undue side-effects.

⚠ Take care if the patient is elderly or in renal failure—consider starting with a ↓ dose of morphine.

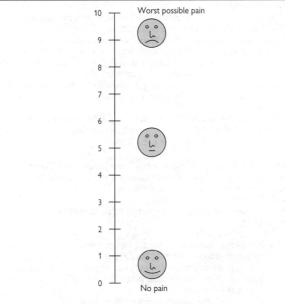

Ask the patient to mark a point on the line that represents their current pain level—where 10 is the worst pain they have ever experienced and 0 is no pain at all.

Fig. 3.2 Simple visual analogue pain scale.

❶ Beware of emergency requests for opioids from patients unknown to you or your practice.

⚠ Diamorphine and morphine are controlled drugs and must be kept in a locked container, stored in a locked car boot or cupboard. Their use must be recorded in a controlled drug register.

Opioid side-effects
- *Nausea and vomiting*—if administering an acute, one-off dose give cyclizine 50 mg IM—unless suspected MI when administer metoclopramide 10 mg IM (as cyclizine can precipitate heart failure). If starting regular opioid medication, anti-emetics, e.g. haloperidol 1.5 mg nocte may be needed short-term (<1 wk). If nausea continues, consider switching to an alternative opioid.
- *Constipation*—consider prescribing prophylactic laxatives, e.g. bisacodyl 1–2 tab nocte if prescribing codeine, morphine or any other opioid on an ongoing basis.
- *Drowsiness/cognitive impairment*—warn about the dangers of driving, performing other skilled tasks and working with dangerous machinery if affected. Usually abates over a few days.

Opioid toxicity: may be increased by dehydration, renal failure, other analgesics (e.g. NSAIDs) and co-administration of amitriptyline. Intentional or unintentional overdose produces:
- Drowsiness or coma
- Confusion—including auditory and/or visual hallucinations
- Vomiting
- Respiratory depression
  - *If respiratory rate ≥8/min and the patient is easily rousable and not cyanosed*—adopt a policy of 'wait and see'. If on regular opioids, consider reducing or omitting the next regular dose of opioid. Stop syringe drivers temporarily to allow plasma levels to ↓, then restart at lower dose.
  - *If respiratory rate <8/min, and the patient is barely rousable/unconscious and/or cyanosed*—if acute opioid overdosage give 0.4–2 mg naloxone IV every 2–3 min until respiratory status is satisfactory to a maximum of 10 mg. If respiratory function still does not improve, question diagnosis. Further boluses may be necessary once respiratory function improves as naloxone is shorter acting than morphine. For those receiving chronic opioids and in palliative care—see 🕮 p.243.
- Pinpoint pupils
- Hypotension
- Muscle rigidity/myoclonus—consider renal failure (can produce myoclonus alone). Treat by rehydration, stopping other medication that may exacerbate myoclonus, switching opioid or with clonazepam 2–4 mg/24 h depending on circumstances.

Addition of co-analgesics and adjuvant drugs: in combination with analgesics, can enhance pain control. Examples include:
- *Antidepressants*—in low dose for nerve pain and sleep disturbance associated with pain (e.g. amitriptyline 10–75 mg nocte); in larger doses for secondary depression (e.g. fluoxetine 20 mg od)
- *Anticonvulsants*—neuropathic pain, e.g. gabapentin—start with 300 mg od on day 1. On day 2 ↑ to 300 mg bd and ↑ again to 300 mg tds on day 3. Increase further according to response to a maximum of 1.8 g daily (in divided doses)

- *Muscle relaxants*—muscle cramp pain, e.g. diazepam 5 mg stat
- *Antispasmodics*—bowel colic, e.g. mebeverine 135 mg tds
- *Antibiotics*—infection pain
- *Night sedative*—when lack of sleep is lowering pain threshold
- *Anxiolytic*—when anxiety is making pain worse.

Clinical scenarios

- *Childhood pain:* treat with paracetamol suspension—120 mg/5ml for children <6 y and 250 mg/5 ml for children >6 y. Add ibuprofen suspension 100 mg/5 ml if analgesia is insufficient.
- *Trauma:* if a patient is in pain and the cause is clear (e.g. fracture), then give opioid and/or non-opioid analgesia. Opioids are contraindicated if there is any suspicion of head injury. Do not give any analgesia if there is any possibility of intra-abdominal injury.
- *Headache:* do not use opioids for pain relief in headache (particularly suspected subarachnoid headache) as opioids might obscure the pupillary reflexes. Migraine frequently responds to IM diclofenac 75 mg ± IM chlorpromazine 25–50 mg. Alternatively consider 5HT1 agonist, e.g. sumatriptan unless 2 injections/tablets/nasal sprays already given in last 24 h (or ergotamine in <24 h)—📖 p.144.
- *Acute abdominal pain:* it is preferable not to give analgesia prior to referring a patient with acute abdominal pain to hospital as this could mask the signs/symptoms important in making the correct diagnosis.
- *Renal colic:* responds well to diclofenac injection. Give 75 mg IM deep into the gluteal muscle. Can be repeated after 30 min either IM or PR. Maximum dose is 150 mg in 24 h.
- *Musculoskeletal pain:* NSAIDs, e.g. ibuprofen 400 mg tds/qds or diclofenac 50 mg tds, 75 mg bd or 100 mg od are useful for analgesia for acute musculoskeletal injuries and exacerbations of arthritic pain.
- *Pain in palliative care:* 📖 p.243.

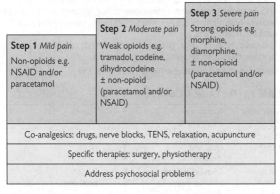

Fig. 3.3 Analgesics ladder.

:O: Coma

Patients in coma/pre-coma nearly always require emergency admission.

When you receive the call for assistance:
- Advise the attendant (unless history of possible spinal injury) to turn the patient on to his/her side
- Call an ambulance to meet you at the scene.

On reaching the patient:
- Assess the need for basic life support:
  - Airways patent?
  - Breathing satisfactory?
  - Circulation adequate?
- Turn into the recovery position (📖 p.30) if no contraindications, e.g. spinal injury.
- Call for ambulance support if you have not already done so.
- Ensure the patient is warm
- Try to establish a diagnosis (see assessment)

As soon as possible:
- Insert an airway
- Give oxygen
- Establish IV access
- Transfer to hospital—unless the condition has resolved, e.g. hypoglycaemia, fit

Possible causes
- *Drugs:* sedatives or hypnotics, opiates, alcohol, solvents, carbon monoxide poisoning.
- *Vascular:* stroke, low cardiac output, e.g. post-MI, ruptured AAA.
- *CNS:* fit or post-ictal state; hydrocephalus (e.g. blocked shunt); cerebral oedema (e.g. meningitis, SAH, head injury); concussion; extradural or subdural haematoma.
- *Metabolic:* hypo- or hyperglycaemia; hypothermia; hypopituitarism.
- *Infection:* meningitis or septicaemia, pneumonia.

Assessment and management (see Figure 3.4)

Table 3.1 The Glasgow Coma Scale

Eye opening:	Spontaneous	4	To pain	2
	To voice	3	None	1
Best verbal response:	Oriented	5	Incomprehensive	2
	Confused	4	None	1
	Inappropriate words	3		
Best motor response:	Obeys command	6	Flexion	3
	Localizes pain	5	Extension	2
	Withdraw	4	None	1

Total score = Eye opening + Best verbal + Best motor response scores.

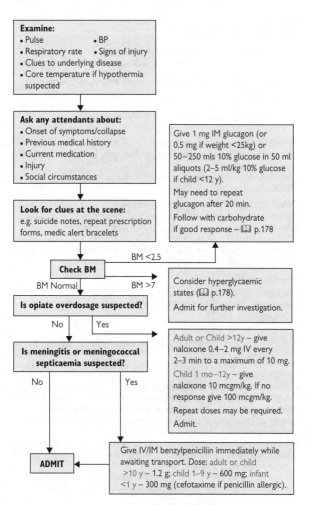

Examine:
- Pulse
- BP
- Respiratory rate
- Signs of injury
- Clues to underlying disease
- Core temperature if hypothermia suspected

Ask any attendants about:
- Onset of symptoms/collapse
- Previous medical history
- Current medication
- Injury
- Social circumstances

Look for clues at the scene:
e.g. suicide notes, repeat prescription forms, medic alert bracelets

Check BM

BM Normal

BM <2.5

BM >7

Give 1 mg IM glucagon (or 0.5 mg if weight <25kg) or 50–250 mls 10% glucose in 50 ml aliquots (2–5 ml/kg 10% glucose if child <12 y).

May need to repeat glucagon after 20 min.

Follow with carbohydrate if good response – 📖 p.178

Consider hyperglycaemic states (📖 p.178).

Admit for further investigation.

Is opiate overdosage suspected?

No   Yes

Is meningitis or meningococcal septicaemia suspected?

No   Yes

Adult or Child >12y – give naloxone 0.4–2 mg IV every 2–3 min to a maximum of 10 mg.

Child 1 mo–12y – give naloxone 10 mcgm/kg. If no response give 100 mcgm/kg.

Repeat doses may be required.

Admit.

ADMIT

Give IV/IM benzylpenicillin immediately while awaiting transport. *Dose:* adult or child >10 y – 1.2 g; child 1–9 y – 600 mg; infant <1 y – 300 mg (cefotaxime if penicillin allergic).

Fig. 3.4 Assessment and management of the unconscious patient.

:O: **Anaphylaxis**

Severe systemic allergic reaction.

Common causes
- *Foods:* nuts, fish and shellfish, sesame seeds and oil, milk, eggs, pulses (beans, peas)
- *Insect stings:* wasp or bee
- *Drugs:* antibiotics, aspirin and other NSAIDs, opiates
- *Latex.*

Essential features: 1 or both of:
- Respiratory difficulty, e.g. wheeze, stridor—may be due to laryngeal oedema or asthma
- Hypotension—can present as fainting, collapse, or loss of consciousness.

Other features: all or some of the following:
- Erythema
- Angio-oedema
- Itching of palate
- Itching of external auditory meatus
- Generalized pruritus
- Rhinitis
- Nausea
- Palpitations
- Urticaria
- Conjunctivitis
- Vomiting
- Sense of impending doom

Examination
- *A*irway—mouth/tongue for oedema
- *B*reathing—Chest (wheeze), PEFR
- *C*irculation—pulse, BP
- *S*kin—check for rashes.

Algorithms for management of anaphylaxis: Figures 3.5 and 3.6—📖 p.46–47.

Follow-up
- Warn patients or parents of the possibility of recurrence.
- Advise sufferers to wear a device (e.g. Medic Alert bracelet) that will inform bystanders or medical staff should a future attack occur.
- Refer all patients after their first anaphylactic attack to a specialist allergy clinic.
- Consider supplying sufferers (or parents) with an EpiPen® or similar that can be used to administer IM epinephrine (adrenaline) immediately should symptoms recur.
- If you supply an EpiPen®, teach anyone likely to need to use it, how to operate the device. Intramuscular epinephrine is very safe.

GP contract: quality points are available for practices that possess the equipment and in-date emergency drugs to treat anaphylaxis (Medicines Indicator 2).

Further information
Resuscitation Council UK Emergency medical treatment of anaphylactic reactions for first medical responders (2005) 🖳 www.resus.org.uk

Action

- If suspected when the initial call for help comes in, call an emergency ambulance immediately—then visit.
- Ask when the initial call is taken if the patient has had a similar event before. If so, ask if he/she has an Epipen or similar. If yes, advise the caller to use it immediately.

On arrival

- Ensure the patient is comfortable—lie down flat ± leg elevation if ↓BP; sit up if breathing difficulty.
- If available, *give oxygen* at high flow rates (10–15 l/min).
- *Give IM adrenaline (epinephrine) to all* patients with clinical signs of shock, airways swelling, or breathing difficulty. *Dose:*
  - Adult or child >12 y: 0.5 ml epinephrine (adrenaline) 1:1000 solution (500 mcgm) IM. Give half dose if: prepubertal or adult on tricyclic antidepressants, monoamine oxidase inhibitors or β blockers.
  - Child 6–12 y: ½ adult dose—0.25 ml of 1:1000 epinephrine (adrenaline) solution (250 mcgm) IM.
  - Child 6 mo–6 y: ¼ adult dose—0.12 ml of 1:1000 epinephrine (adrenaline) solution (120 mcgm) IM.
  - Child <6 mo: 0.05 ml 1:1000 epinephrine (adrenaline) solution (50 mcgm) IM. Absolute accuracy of dose is not necessary.
- *Repeat* after ≥5 min if improvement is transient, no improvement or deterioration after initial treatment. May need several doses.
- *Give an antihistamine:* Dose of chlorphenamine:
  - Adults and children >12 y—10–20 mg IM
  - Children 6–12 y—5–10 mg IM
  - Children 1–6 y—2.5–5 mg IM
- *Give hydrocortisone* by IM or slow IV injection. *Dose:*
  - Adults and children >12 y—100–500 mg
  - Children 6–11 y—100 mg
  - Children 1–6 y—50 mg
  - Children <1 y—25 mg
- *Give salbutamol* if bronchospasm.
- If severe hypotension does not respond rapidly, start an IV infusion (if available) and *rapidly infuse 1–2 l of saline until BP* ↑(children 20 ml/kg rapidly then another similar dose if not responding).
- *Admit the patient to hospital* until ill effects have settled.

❶ The preferred site for IM injection is the midpoint of the anterolateral thigh

---

Information and support for patients
Allergy UK ☎ 01322 619898 ▭ www.allergyuk.org
Anaphylaxis Campaign ☎ 01252 542029 ▭ www.anaphylaxis.org.uk
Medic Alert Foundation Supply Medic Alert bracelets. ☎ 0800 581 420
▭ www.medicalert.co.uk

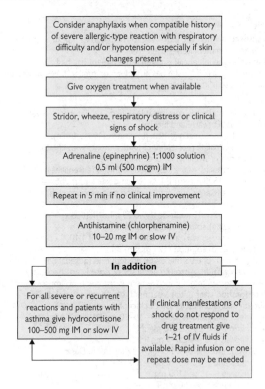

Fig. 3.5 Anaphylactic reactions: treatment algorithm for adults.

Figures 3.5 and 3.6 are reproduced with permission of Resuscitation Council (UK)

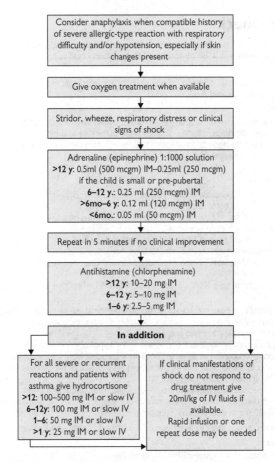

Fig. 3.6 Anaphylactic reactions: treatment algorithm for children.

☼ Shock

Shock is due to inadequate blood flow to the peripheral circulation. It usually results in ↓ BP (± tachycardia), peripheral cyanosis, and ↓ urinary output.

Hypovolaemic shock: usually due to haemorrhage, e.g. GI bleeding (📖 p.50), ruptured AAA (📖 p.52).

Signs
- *Initially*—tachycardia (pulse >100 bpm), pallor, sweating ± restlessness
- *Later*—decompensation—sudden fall in pulse rate and BP. Young people may decompensate very rapidly—if tachycardic treat as a medical emergency—speed could be life saving.

Action
- Lie the patient down flat and raise legs above waist height.
- Call for ambulance assistance.
- Control bleeding by applying pressure if obvious bleeding point (e.g. nose bleed, laceration).
- Gain IV access and (if possible) take blood for FBC and cross-matching—try to insert 2 large bore cannulae.
- If available, start plasma expander/IV fluids. Give rapidly over 10–15 min.
- If available give 100% oxygen—unless COPD when give 24%.

Terminally ill patients: bleeding can be a terminal event in patients with cancer. Where possible, make a decision in advance about whether to treat severe bleeding and prepare carers.
- *If a decision is made to treat*—treat as for hypovolaemic shock and admit to hospital as an emergency. ❶ if bleeding from a lung tumour, protect the airways and lie the patient on the side of the tumour to protect the healthy lung.
- *If a decision is made not to treat*—stay with the patient and give sedative medication (e.g. midazolam 20–40 mg s/cut or IV, or diazepam 10–20 mg pr ± analgesia). Support the carers.

Cardiogenic shock: heart pump failure, e.g. MI, arrhythmia, tamponade.

Signs
- Hypotension—systolic BP <80–90 mmHg
- Pulse rate may be normal, ↑ or ↓
- Severe breathlessness ± cyanosis.

Action
- Sit the patient up if possible
- Call for ambulance assistance
- Treat any underlying cause found, e.g. atropine for bradycardia; diamorphine, furosemide and GTN spray (if tolerated) for acute LVF
- Gain IV access if possible
- If available give 100% oxygen—unless COPD when give 24%.

Septic shock: due to toxins from bacterial infection, e.g. meningitis.

Signs
- Hypotension
- Tachycardia
- Peripheral vasodilation or shut down (peripheral pallor and cyanosis, cool extremities)
- Pyrexia
- Tachypnoea
- ± purpuric rash

Action
- Lie the patient down flat and raise legs above waist height
- Call for ambulance assistance
- Give IV/IM benzylpenicillin immediately while awaiting transport. *Dose:*
  - Adult and child ≥10 y—1.2 g
  - Child 1–9 y—600 mg
  - Infant <1 y—300 mg.
- If possible gain IV access while awaiting the ambulance and take blood for cultures.
- If available, start plasma expander/IV fluids. Give rapidly over 10–15 min.
- If available, give 100% oxygen—unless COPD when give 24%.

Anaphylactic shock: 📖 p.44–47.

Other rarer causes of shock: Admit as medical emergencies:
- *Neurogenic*—due to cerebral trauma or haemorrhage, e.g. head injury, subarachnoid haemorrhage
- *Poisoning*
- *Liver failure*.

:O: Bleeding

Seriousness depends on the site and amount of bleeding, and type of blood vessels damaged. Adults have ~5 l of blood and can safely lose ½ l. but rapid loss of larger volumes results in hypovolaemic shock and death.

⚠ Beware of HIV/hepatitis risk from blood contact (📖 p.157)

❶ Young people can lose a lot of blood before their BP drops: be worried if a young person is tachycardic. Tachycardia may not develop in patients on β-blockers

Hypovolaemic shock: 📖 p.48.

Bleeding external wounds: apply pressure to the wound. If the wound is on a limb, elevate the limb. If the bleeding does not stop and/or if further treatment is required which cannot be done in the community (e.g. suturing), transfer to A&E.

Gastrointestinal (GI) bleeding: take all GI bleeds seriously. Fatal in ~1:10 elderly patients admitted to hospital.

Causes of GI bleeding

Upper GI bleed:
- Peptic ulcer
- Gastritis
- Mallory–Weiss tear
- Oesophagitis
- Oesophageal or gastric cancer
- Oesophageal varices
- Drugs—steroids, anticoagulants, NSAIDs
- Angiodysplasia
- Haemangioma
- Bleeding disorders
- Swallowed blood from nosebleed

Lower GI bleed:
- Diverticulitis
- Colitis—infectious/inflammatory
- Large bowel tumour or polyp
- Haemorrhoids
- Anal fissure
- Angiodysplasia (arteriovenous malformations are common)
- Haemangioma
- Bleeding disorders
- Blood from upper GI bleed

Risk factors

Upper GI bleed:
- History of alcohol abuse
- History of chronic liver disease
- History of NSAID use
- History of oral steroid use

Lower GI bleed:
- Change in bowel habit
- History of diverticulitis
- History of UC

All GI bleeds:
- Anticoagulant use
- Serious medical conditions (e.g. cardiovascular, respiratory or renal disease)
- Recent tiredness (? due to anaemia).

Presentation
Upper GI bleeding: typical presentation:
- Haematemesis—vomiting of blood
- Melaena—passage of black, offensive, tarry stool consisting of digested blood per rectum. ❶ Iron tablets may cause black stools.

Lower GI bleeding: passage of fresh blood PR ❶ Very heavy upper GI bleeds can present with fresh red bleeding PR.

Other features that may be present (and may precede bleeding):
- Faintness or dizziness especially on standing
- Patient feels cold or clammy
- Collapse ± cardiac arrest.

Examination
- Colour—pallor, peripheral cyanosis
- Pulse—tachycardia
- BP—↓ and/or postural drop
- JVP—↓
- Vomitus

Immediate action
- When the call for help is received—arrange immediate emergency transfer of the patient to hospital if a significant acute GI bleed is suspected.
- Attend the patient if diagnosis from history is unclear or (if possible) once the ambulance has been called to assist
- Regard as an emergency until proved otherwise.

On arrival: briefly assess the severity of the bleed from history and examination. If a significant GI bleed is suspected:
- Lie the patient flat and lift legs higher than body (e.g. feet on a pillow).
- Insert a large bore IV cannula—the opportunity may be lost by the time the ambulance crew arrive. If possible take a sample for FBC and X-match on insertion.
- If available, give oxygen.
- If available start plasma expander/IV fluids.
- Transfer as rapidly as possible to hospital.

Coffee-grounds vomit
- Vomiting of altered blood—looks like coffee granules.
- Implies upper GI bleeding—though less severe than fresh red blood.
- History and examination as for acute GI bleed.
- Always admit to hospital for further assessment.

Management in terminally ill patients: if a terminally ill patient has a severe, life-threatening bleed, make a decision whether the cause of the bleed is treatable or a terminal event. This is best done in advance but bleeding can't always be predicted.
- *If active treatment is indicated*—treat as for acute GI bleeding (above).
- *If no active treatment is indicated:*
  - Stay with the patient
  - Give sedative medication, e.g. midazolam 20–40 mg s/cut or IV or diazepam 10–20 mg pr ± analgesia
  - Support carers as big bleeds are extremely distressing.

❶ Unless a patient is very near to death, admit all non-life-threatening GI bleeds. Palliative treatment options include laser treatment and arterial embolization—both can be performed on frail patients.

Bleeding aneurysm

Ruptured abdominal aortic aneurysm (AAA)

- In the community setting, death rate from ruptured AAA ≈90% (80% die before reaching hospital and 50% that get to hospital die during surgery).
- Consider a ruptured AAA in any patient with ↓BP and atypical abdominal symptoms (especially if there is a pulsatile abdominal mass).

△ In a patient with a known AAA, abdominal pain represents a ruptured AAA unless proven otherwise.

Dissecting thoracic aneurysm: typically presents with sudden tearing chest pain radiating to the back. Consider in any patient with ↓BP and chest pain especially if pain radiates through to the back. As dissection progresses, branches of the aorta are sequentially occluded causing:

- hemiplegia—carotid artery
- unequal pulses and BP in the two arms—subclavian artery
- paraplegia—spinal arteries
- acute renal failure—renal arteries.

Proximal extension may cause aortic incompetence and MI (cardiac arteries).

Action

- Obtain venous access with 2× large bore IV cannulae.
- Admit as 'blue light' emergency keeping the patient flat in the ambulance.
- Warn relatives of poor prognosis.

Nose bleed/epistaxis: epistaxis (or nose bleed) is usually due to ruptured blood vessels on the nasal septum (most commonly the vein behind the comella or Little's area).

Causes

- *Elderly:* degenerative arterial disease, ↑ BP, nose picking, coryza, allergic rhinitis, medication (warfarin or aspirin), blood dyscrasias, teleangiectasia and tumours. Often no cause is found.
- *Young:* nose picking, coryza, allergic rhinitis, blood dyscrasias.

Action: Figure 3.4.

Hospital management

- Anterior nasal packing using ribbon gauze impregnated with paraffin or a nasal tampon. The pack is usually left in place for 24 h.
- Posterior nasal packing, e.g. using a Foley catheter.
- Blood transfusion—rarely needed.
- Surgical exploration—occasionally required to find and cauterize the bleeding point or ligate the bleeding artery.

Recurrent minor nosebleeds: refer routinely to ENT.

Very heavy menstrual bleeding: p.183.

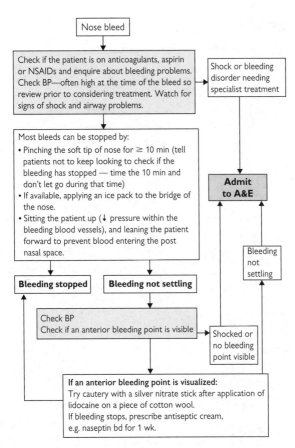

Fig. 3.7 Acute management of nosebleed in the community.

Cardiovascular emergencies

☼ Chest pain

Chest pain is a common symptom.

⚠ Always think—could this be an MI, PE, dissecting aneurysm, or pericarditis?

On receiving the call for assistance

Ask:
- Nature and location of the pain?
- Duration of the pain?
- Other associated symptoms—sweating, nausea, shortness of breath, palpitations?
- Past medical history (particularly heart disease, high cholesterol)?
- Family history (particularly heart disease)?
- Smoker?

Action
- Consider differential diagnosis (Table 4.1)
- If MI is suspected call for ambulance assistance before (or instead of) visiting.
- Otherwise arrange surgery appointment, or visit, as appropriate, assess and treat according to cause.

Further assessment

History: ask about:
- Site and nature of pain. Any history of trauma?
- Duration
- Associated symptoms (e.g. breathlessness, nausea)
- Provoking and relieving factors
- PMH, FH (e.g. heart disease), drug history, smoking history.

Examination
- Check BP in both arms
- General appearance—distress, sweating, pallor
- JVP and carotid pulse
- Respiratory rate
- Apex beat
- Heart sounds
- Lung fields
- Local tenderness
- Pain on movement of chest
- Skin rashes
- Swelling or tenderness of legs (?DVT).

Investigations: ECG and CXR may be helpful.

⚠ Refer any patient with unexplained chest/shoulder pain of >3 wk duration for urgent CXR.

Further information

NICE Referral guidelines for suspected cancer—quick reference guide (2005) ▣ www.nice.org.uk

Table 4.1 Causes of acute chest pain

Diagnosis	Features
MI 📖 p.58	Band like chest pain around the chest or central chest pressure/dull ache ± radiation to shoulders, arms (L>R), neck and/or jaw. Often associated with nausea, sweating and/or shortness of breath.
Unstable angina	As for MI
Pericarditis	Sharp, constant sternal pain relieved by sitting forwards. May radiate to left shoulder ± arm or into the abdomen. Worse lying on the left side and on inspiration, swallowing and coughing.
Dissecting thoracic aneurysm 📖 p.52	Typically presents with sudden tearing chest pain radiating to the back. Consider in any patient with chest pain and ↓ BP—especially if pain radiates through to the back.
PE 📖 p.80	Acute dyspnoea, sharp chest pain (worse on inspiration), haemoptysis and/or syncope. Tachycardic and mild pyrexia.
Pleurisy 📖 p.84	Sharp, localized chest pain, worse on inspiration. May be associated with symptoms and signs of a chest infection.
Pneumothorax 📖 p.81	Sudden onset of pleuritic chest pain or ↑ breathlessness ± pallor and tachycardia.
Oesophageal spasm, oesophagitis	Central chest pain. May be associated with acid reflux (though not always). May be described as burning but often indistinguishable from cardiac pain. May respond to antacids.
Musculoskeletal pain	Localized pain—worse on movement. May be a history of injury
Shingles	Intense, often sharp, unilateral pain. Responds poorly to analgesia. May be present several days before rash appears.
Costochondritis	Inflammation of the costochondral junctions—tenderness over the costochondral junction and pain in the affected area on springing the chest wall.
Bornholm's disease	Unilateral chest and/or abdominal pain, rhinitis. Coxsackie virus infection. Treat with simple analgesia.
Idiopathic chest pain	No cause apparent. Common. Affects young people >elderly people. ♀>♂

⚠ If a patient is acutely unwell with chest pain and the cause is not clear, err on the side of caution and admit for further assessment

☼ Myocardial infarct and unstable angina

⚠ Diagnosis of myocardial infarct (MI) is sometimes not obvious: always have a high index of suspicion.

Typical presentation: sustained central chest pain not relieved by sublingual GTN.

Other features that may be present:
● Collapse ± cardiac arrest
● Breathlessness
● Anxiety/fear of dying
● Nausea ± vomiting
● Sweating
● Pain in 1 or both arms, jaw, back or upper abdomen.

❶ May occasionally be silent especially in patients with DM.

Examination: pulse, BP, JVP, heart sounds, chest (?pulmonary oedema)

Investigation: *ECG*—ST elevation (Figure 4.1) *or* R waves and ST depression in leads V1–V3 (posterior infarction) *or* new LBBB.

> **Action**
>
> *When the call for assistance is made:* if MI is suspected, arrange immediate transfer to hospital—for thrombolysis to be effective it must be given as soon as possible after the onset of pain. Seeing the patient before arranging transfer introduces unnecessary delays.
>
> If possible attend the patient once the ambulance has been called to assist—there is a lot a GP can do that an ambulance crew cannot. If the patient is seen:
> ● give aspirin 300 mg po (unless contraindicated)
> ● insert IV cannula
> ● give IV analgesia (e.g. morphine 2.5–5 mg). Repeat in 15 min as necessary
> ● give IV antiemetic (metoclopramide 10 mg)
> ● give sublingual GTN to act as a coronary artery vasodilator if systolic BP >90 and pulse <100 bpm
> ● if available, give oxygen
> ● if bradycardia give atropine 300 mcgm IV and further doses of 300 mcgm if needed to a maximum of 1.2 mg.
>
> *Thrombolysis in general practice:* may be appropriate in places where transfer to hospital takes >½ h. Special training and equipment is necessary.

Late calls
- *If the patient is seen <24 h after an acute episode:* admit for specialist assessment.
- *If the patient is seen >24 h after an acute episode but still has residual pain or other symptoms:* admit.
- *If the patient is seen >24 h after an acute episode and is well,* start regular aspirin, supply with GTN spray, and warn to call for assistance (by calling ambulance and/or emergency GP) if chest pain lasts >20 min despite GTN spray. Refer to cardiology for follow-up.

Unstable angina: pain on minimal or no exertion, pain at rest (may occur at night) or angina which is rapidly worsening in intensity, frequency or duration. 15% suffer MI in <1 mo.

Management: it is often difficult to tell the difference between acute myocardial infarct (MI) and unstable angina in general practice. Treat as for acute MI and admit if attacks are severe, occur at rest or last >20 min even with GTN spray.

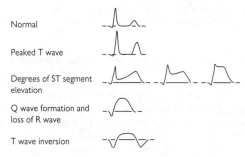

Normal

Peaked T wave

Degrees of ST segment elevation

Q wave formation and loss of R wave

T wave inversion

Fig. 4.1 Sequence of ECG changes after MI.

Fig. 4.1 is reproduced from ABC of clinical electrocardiography (ISBN: 0727915363) with permission from BMJ Publishing.

Tachycardia

⊚ **Palpitations:** the uncomfortable awareness of heart beat. Can be physiological (e.g. after exercise, at times of stress) or signify arrhythmia. Can cause a feeling of faintness or even collapse (e.g. Stokes–Adams attack, due to AV block) Ask the patient to tap out the rhythm.

⊚ **Tachycardia:** heart rate >100 bpm. The patient may experience the sensation of rapid, irregular or forceful heart beats. Common and may be an incidental finding. History and examination can exclude significant problems in most patients.

History: ask about:
- *Palpitations*—duration, frequency and pattern, rhythm
- *Precipitating/relieving factors*
- *Associated symptoms*—chest pain, collapse or funny turns, sweating, breathlessness or hyperventilation
- *Past history*, e.g. previous episodes, heart disease, thyroid disease
- *Lifestyle*—drug history; caffeine/alcohol intake; smoking.

⚠ **Red flag symptoms**
- Pre-existing cardiovascular disease
- FH of syncope, arrhythmia or sudden death
- Arrhythmia associated with falls and/or syncope

Examination
- *General examination*—for anaemia, thyrotoxicosis, anxiety, other systemic disease
- *Cardiovascular examination*—heart size, pulse rate and rhythm, JVP, BP, heart sounds and murmurs, evidence of left ventricular failure.

Investigations: if the patient is well and the palpitations have settled, investigation can be delayed. If the tachycardia is ongoing or the patient is unwell, investigate immediately with a resting ECG.

Further investigations: if ECG is abnormal or other concerning features:
- Ambulatory ECG or cardiac memo
- Echo if <50 y or murmur/left ventricular failure detected
- Exercise tolerance test if exercise related
- *Blood:* TFTs, FBC, ESR, U&E, fasting blood glucose, Ca^{2+}, albumin.

No tachycardia and no ECG abnormalities: reassure. Explore the possibility of anxiety disorder.

:⚙: **Ventricular tachycardia (VT):** broad (>3 small squares) QRS complexes at a rate of >100 bpm on ECG (Figure 4.2)

Management
- Admit as blue light emergency.
- Meanwhile give O_2 if available ± 100 mg IV lidocaine.
- If no pulse treat as VF cardiac arrest (▢ p.22)

⊛ **Ventricular ectopic beats:** additional broad QRS complexes, without p-waves, superimposed on regular sinus rhythm (Figure 4.4). Usually felt by the patient as 'missed beats'. Common and usually of no clinical significance. Rarely may be the presenting feature of viral myocarditis.

Management

- *Frequent ectopics (>100/h) on ECG:* refer urgently to cardiology.
- *R on T phenomenon on ECG:* rarely ectopics can cause ventricular fibrillation—particularly if coinciding with the T wave of a preceding beat ('R on T phenomenon'—Figure 4.5). If occurs >10×/min—admit.
- *After MI:* ventricular extrasystoles after MI are associated with ↑ mortality. Refer to cardiology.
- *No sinister features on ECG:* explain the benign nature of the condition. Advise avoidance of caffeine, alcohol, smoking and fatigue. β blockers can be helpful for patients unable to tolerate ectopics despite reassurance.

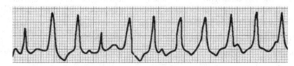

Fig. 4.2 Ventricular tachycardia.

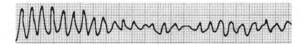

Fig. 4.3 Ventricular fibrillation.

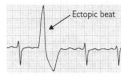

Ectopic beat

Fig. 4.4 Ventricular ectopic beat.

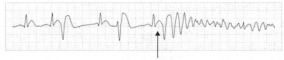

Ectopic beat coinciding with T provoking a run of VF

Fig. 4.5 R on T phenomenon.

Figure 4.2 is reproduced from the ABC of clinical electrocardiography with permission from BMJ publishing.

ⓔ **Sinus tachycardia:** consider infection, pain, MI, shock, exercise, emotion (including anxiety), heart failure, thyrotoxicosis, drugs.

⚠ **Paroxysmal supraventricular tachycardia (SVT):** narrow QRS complex tachycardia with a regular rate >100 bpm on ECG (Figure 4.6).

Management

If seen during an attack:
- Get an ECG if possible
- Try carotid sinus massage (unless elderly, IHD, digoxin toxic, carotid bruit, history of TIAs), the Valsalva manoeuvre and/or ice on the face (especially effective for children).
- Admit as an emergency if the attack continues.
- If the attack stops, refer to cardiology for advice on further management enclosing a copy of the ECG trace during an attack if available.

If diagnosed from history or ambulatory ECG trace: refer to cardiology for confirmation of diagnosis and initiation of treatment—urgent referral if chest pain, dizziness or breathlessness during attacks. Enclose the ECG trace during an attack if available.

Treatment options are: sotalol, verapamil or amiodarone.

Advice: advise patients to avoid caffeine, alcohol and smoking.

⚠ **Atrial fibrillation:** common disturbance of cardiac rhythm that may be episodic (*paroxysmal*) or chronic. Characterized by rapid irregularly irregular narrow QRS complex tachycardia with absence of P-waves (Figure 4.7). Associated with 5× ↑ risk of stroke. Acute AF may be precipitated by acute infection, high alcohol intake, surgery, electrocution, MI, pericarditis, PE or hyperthyroidism.

Symptoms: often asymptomatic but may cause palpitations, chest pain, stroke/TIA, dyspnoea, fatigue, lightheadedness and/or syncope.

Examination
- *General examination:* check for anaemia, thyrotoxicosis, anxiety, and other systemic disease
- *Cardiovascular examination:* check heart size, pulse rate and rhythm (apex rate >radial pulse rate when a patient is in AF), JVP, BP, heart sounds and murmurs, and for evidence of left ventricular failure.

Management: Figure 4.9, 🕮 p.64.

Further information: atrial fibrillation: the management of atrial fibrillation (NICE, 2006) 🖥 www.nice.org.uk

⚠ **Atrial flutter:** ECG shows regular saw-tooth baseline at rate of 300 bpm with a narrow QRS complex tachycardia superimposed at a rate of 150 bpm or 100 bpm (Figure 4.8). Manage in the same way as AF (though specialist drug treatment may differ).

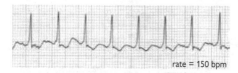

Fig. 4.6 Paroxysmal SVT.

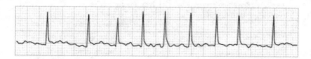

- Irregular rate and rhythm
- No P waves + irregular baseline
- Irregular QRS complexes

Fig. 4.7 ECG from a patient with atrial fibrillation.

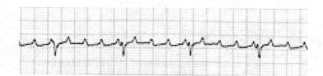

- Regular saw-tooth baseline at rate 300 bpm
- QRS complexes at rate of 100 bpm

Fig. 4.8 ECG from a patient with atrial flutter.

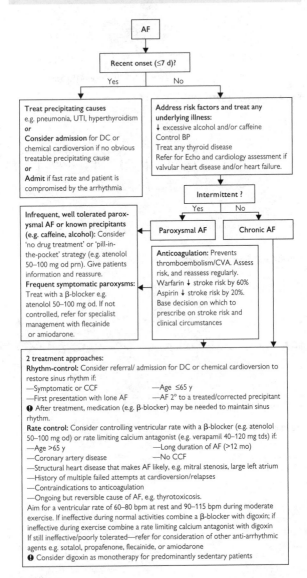

AF

Recent onset (≤7 d)?

Yes — No

Yes:

Treat precipitating causes
e.g. pneumonia, UTI, hyperthyroidism
or
Consider admission for DC or chemical cardioversion if no obvious treatable precipitating cause
or
Admit if fast rate and patient is compromised by the arrhythmia

No:

Address risk factors and treat any underlying illness:
↓ excessive alcohol and/or caffeine
Control BP
Treat any thyroid disease
Refer for Echo and cardiology assessment if valvular heart disease and/or heart failure.

Intermittent ?

Yes — No

Paroxysmal AF — **Chronic AF**

Infrequent, well tolerated paroxysmal AF or known precipitants (e.g. caffeine, alcohol): Consider 'no drug treatment' or 'pill-in-the-pocket' strategy (e.g. atenolol 50–100 mg od prn). Give patients information and reassure.
Frequent symptomatic paroxysms:
Treat with a β-blocker e.g. atenolol 50–100 mg od. If not controlled, refer for specialist management with flecainide or amiodarone.

Anticoagulation: Prevents thromboembolism/CVA. Assess risk, and reassess regularly.
Warfarin ↓ stroke risk by 60%
Aspirin ↓ stroke risk by 20%.
Base decision on which to prescribe on stroke risk and clinical circumstances

2 treatment approaches:
Rhythm-control: Consider referral/ admission for DC or chemical cardioversion to restore sinus rhythm if:
—Symptomatic or CCF   —Age ≤65 y
—First presentation with lone AF   —AF 2° to a treated/corrected precipitant
❶ After treatment, medication (e.g. β-blocker) may be needed to maintain sinus rhythm.
Rate control: Consider controlling ventricular rate with a β-blocker (e.g. atenolol 50–100 mg od) or rate limiting calcium antagonist (e.g. verapamil 40–120 mg tds) if:
—Age >65 y   —Long duration of AF (>12 mo)
—Coronary artery disease   —No CCF
—Structural heart disease that makes AF likely, e.g. mitral stenosis, large left atrium
—History of multiple failed attempts at cardioversion/relapses
—Contraindications to anticoagulation
—Ongoing but reversible cause of AF, e.g. thyrotoxicosis.
Aim for a ventricular rate of 60–80 bpm at rest and 90–115 bpm during moderate exercise. If ineffective during normal activities combine a β-blocker with digoxin; if ineffective during exercise combine a rate limiting calcium antagonist with digoxin
If still ineffective/poorly tolerated—refer for consideration of other anti-arrhythmic agents e.g. sotalol, propafenone, flecainide, or amiodarone
❶ Consider digoxin as monotherapy for predominantly sedentary patients

Fig. 4.9 Management of AF in primary care.

🔔 Bradycardia

Heart rate <60 bpm.

Presentation: often an incidental finding but may present with faints or blackouts, drop attacks, dizziness, breathlessness, or lack of energy.

Examination: slow pulse rate; normal or low BP ± evidence of 2° heart failure. There may also be symptoms/signs of associated disease.

Investigations

- *ECG:* see Fig. 4.10–4.12; ambulatory ECG may help with diagnosis of intermittent bradycardia (e.g. sick sinus syndrome)
- *Blood:* TFTs, FBC, ESR, U&E, LFTs, digoxin levels (if taking digoxin).

Sinus bradycardia: constant bradycardia. P-waves present and P–R interval <0.2 sec (1 large square)—Figure 4.10. *Causes:*

- Physiological, e.g. athletes
- Vasovagal attack
- Drugs, e.g. β blockers, digoxin
- Inferior MI
- Sick sinus syndrome
- Hypothyroidism
- Hypothermia
- ↑ ICP
- Jaundice

Management: admit acutely if symptomatic. Refer for cardiology opinion if asymptomatic but HR <40 bpm or pauses of >3 sec on ECG, despite treatment of reversible causes.

AV node block (heart block): *causes:*

- IHD
- Drugs (digoxin, verapamil)
- Myocarditis
- Cardiomyopathy
- Fibrosis
- Lyme disease (rare)

Types of heart block

- *1st degree block:* fixed P–R interval >200 ms (1 large square); Figure 4.11.
- *2nd degree block:*
  - *Mobitz type I* (Wenckebach)—progressively lengthening P–R interval followed by a dropped beat; Figure 4.12
  - *Mobitz type II*—constant P–R interval with regular dropped beats (e.g. 2:1—every 2nd beat is dropped—consider drug toxicity); Figure 4.12.
- *3rd degree block* (complete heart block): P–P intervals are constant and R–R intervals are constant but not related to each other; Figure 4.13.

Management: untreated 2nd and 3rd degree heart block have a mortality of ≈35%. Refer all patients to cardiology even if asymptomatic. If symptomatic (↓BP <90 mmHg systolic, left ventricular failure, heart rate <40 bpm) admit as an emergency—give IV atropine and O₂ (if available) while awaiting admission.

Stokes–Adams attacks: cardiac arrest due to AV block. Results in sudden loss of consciousness ± some limb twitching due to cerebral anoxia. The patient becomes pale and pulseless but respiration continues. Attacks usually last ~30 sec though occasionally are fatal. On recovery the patient becomes flushed. Refer to cardiology if suspected.

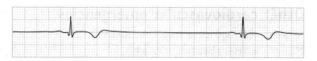

Fig. 4.10 Sinus bradycardia.

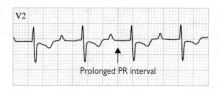

Fig. 4.11 1st degree heart block.

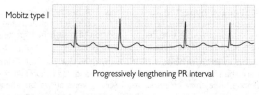

Fig. 4.12 2nd degree heart block.

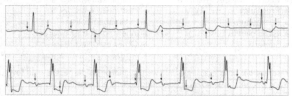

P–P interval and R–R interval are constant but not related to each other
(P waves are marked)

Fig. 4.13 3rd degree (complete) heart block.

Figures 4.11–4.13 are reproduced from the *ABC of clinical electrocardiography* with permission from BMJ Publishing.

Other cardiovascular emergencies

⊚ **Acute left ventricular failure (acute LVF):** 📖 p.78.

Mesenteric artery ischaemia: 📖 p.104.

⊛ **Acute limb ischaemia**

Causes
- Acute thrombotic occlusion of pre-existing stenotic segment (60%)
- Embolus (30%)
- Trauma, e.g. compartment syndrome or traumatic vessel damage

Presentation
- Pain
- Pallor
- Paraesthesia
- Pulselessness
- Paralysis
- Perishing cold

Management: admit under the care of a vascular surgeon. Treatment can be surgical (e.g. embolectomy) or medical (e.g. thrombolysis).

⊛ **Malignant hypertension:** *presents with* headache, very elevated BP (diastolic >140 mmHg), renal failure, fits, coma (encephalopathy), and severe retinopathy. Life-threatening condition. If malignant hypertension is suspected admit as an acute medical emergency.

⊚ **Deep vein thrombosis (DVT):** any deep vein can clot. Common sites are the limbs, mesentery, cerebral sinus and retina. DVT in the leg (commonest site) may be proximal—involving veins above the knee—or isolated to the calf veins. *Incidence:* 1:1000 people/y. in developed countries.

Box 4.1 Risk factors for DVT

- Age ≥ 40 y
- Smoking
- Obesity
- Immobility
- Recent long distance travel
- Pregnancy
- Puerperium
- COC pill/HRT use
- Surgery
- Recent trauma
- Malignancy
- Heart failure
- Nephrotic syndrome
- Inflammatory bowel disease
- Past medical history of thromboembolism
- Inherited clotting disorder
- Other chronic illness

Presentation: unilateral leg pain, swelling and/or tenderness ± mild fever, pitting oedema, warmth and distended collateral superficial veins.

Differential diagnosis
- Cellulitis
- Haematoma
- Ruptured Baker's cyst
- Superficial thrombophlebitis
- Chronic venous insufficiency
- Venous obstruction
- Post-thrombotic syndrome
- Acute arterial ischaemia
- Lymphoedema
- Fracture
- Hypoproteinaemia

Immediate action: clinical diagnosis is unreliable.
- Only 50% of DVTs are symptomatic
- <50% with clinically suspected DVT have diagnosis confirmed.
- ❶ Refer all suspected DVTs for further assessment. Many hospitals have rapid access to facilities for diagnosis, bypassing conventional admission.

☺ **Simple faint/vasovagal attack:** common. Peripheral vasodilation, bradycardia and venous pooling → postural hypotension. Often cause is unclear though ♀>♂. *Known precipitants:* fright (e.g. during venesection) or emotion.

Diagnosis: a typical attack takes following pattern:
- *Prodromal symptoms*—nausea, clammy sweating, blurring, greying and possible loss of vision, lightheadedness, dizziness and tinnitus, yawning. The collection is characteristic.
- *Anoxic phase*—loss of consciousness, pallor, sweating, pupil dilatation, tachypnoea, bradycardia. Muscle tone is ↓, causing eyes to roll up, and the patient to fall. There may be myoclonic jerks as the patient falls.
- *Recovery*—in the horizontal position, skin colour, pulse and consciousness usually return within seconds. ❶ If the patient is unable to fall and is kept upright a 2° anoxic seizure may occur.
- *After-effects*—confusion, amnesia and drowsiness are not prolonged. Injury and incontinence are rare but may occur. Tongue biting is very rare.

Presyncope: term applied to a less severe attack with partial loss of consciousness and a near fall.

Management: exclude other reasons for loss of consciousness. Reassure the patient.

Respiratory emergencies

☼ The choking adult

⚠ If blockage of the airway is only partial, the victim will usually be able to dislodge the foreign body by coughing. If obstruction is complete urgent intervention is required to prevent asphyxia.

Is foreign body airways obstruction (FBAO) likely?
- Sudden onset of respiratory distress while eating?
- Is the victim clutching his neck?

Is the patient coughing effectively?
Signs of an effective cough include:
- In response to the question '*Are you choking?*' the victim answers and says 'Yes'
- Fully responsive—able to speak, cough and breathe
- ▶▶ *Encourage the victim to cough and monitor*

Signs of an ineffective cough include:
- In response to the question '*Are you choking?* ' the victim either responds by nodding or is unable to respond
- Breathing sounds wheezy
- Unable to breathe
- Attempts at coughing are silent
- Unconscious
- ▶▶ *Call for assistance (e.g. dial 999) and assess conscious level*

If victim IS conscious but has absent/ineffective coughing:
- Give up to 5 back blows as needed
- If back blows don't relieve the obstruction, give up to 5 abdominal thrusts as needed.

Following back blows, or abdominal thrusts: reassess:

If the object has not been expelled and the victim is still conscious: continue the sequence of back blows and abdominal thrusts.

If the object is expelled successfully: assess clinical condition (including abdominal examination if abdominal thrusts used). If there is any suspicion part of the object is still in the respiratory tract or there are any intra-abdominal injuries as a result of abdominal thrusts, refer to A&E for assessment.

If the victim becomes UNCONSCIOUS:
- Support the victim carefully to the ground
- Immediately call an ambulance
- Begin CPR (📖 p.18) with 30 chest compressions at a rate of 100/min—even if carotid pulse is present

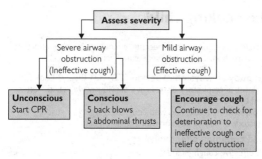

Fig. 5.1 Algorithm for the management of choking in adults.

Back blows for adults

- Stand to the side and slightly behind the victim
- Support the chest with 1 hand and lean the victim well forwards so that when the obstructing object is dislodged it comes out of the mouth
- Give up to 5 sharp blows between the shoulder blades with the heel of the other hand.

Abdominal thrusts for adults

- Stand behind the victim and put both arms around the upper part of the abdomen
- Lean the victim forwards
- Clench your fist and place it between the umbilicus and bottom end of the sternum
- Grasp this hand with your other hand and pull sharply inwards and upwards. Repeat up to 5 times as needed.

Foreign body in the throat: occurs after eating—fish bone or food bolus are most common. Can cause severe discomfort, distress and inability to swallow saliva.

Management: refer immediately to A&E or ENT for investigation (lateral neck X-ray ± laryngoscopy). Most fish bones have passed and the discomfort comes from mucosal trauma. Food boluses often pass spontaneously (especially if the patient is given a smooth muscle relaxant) but occasionally need removal under GA.

Further information

Resuscitation Council (UK) 🖳 www.resus.org.uk

☼ The choking child

⚠ If the child is breathing spontaneously, encourage his own efforts to clear the obstruction. ONLY intervene if ineffective.

Is foreign body airways obstruction (FBAO) likely? Look for:
- Sudden onset of respiratory distress in a previously well child—often witnessed by the child's carer
- Respiratory distress associated with coughing, gagging or stridor
- Recent history of playing with or eating small objects.

Is the child coughing effectively?

Signs of an effective cough include:
- Fully responsive—crying or verbal response to questions
- Loud cough and able to take a breath before coughing.
- ▶▶ *Encourage the child to cough and monitor*

Signs of an ineffective cough include:
- Unable to vocalize
- Quiet or silent cough
- Unable to breathe ± cyanosis
- Decreasing level of consciousness.
- ▶▶ *Call for assistance (e.g. dial 999) and assess conscious level*

If the child IS conscious but has absent/ineffective coughing: give up to 5 back blows as needed. If back blows don't relieve the obstruction, give up to 5 chest thrusts (infants <1 y) *or* up to 5 abdominal thrusts (children ≥1 y) as needed. Then reassess:
- *If the object has not been expelled and the victim is still conscious:* continue the sequence of back blows and chest (for infant) or abdominal (for children) thrusts. ❶ Don't leave the child
- *If the object is expelled successfully:* assess clinical condition (including abdominal examination if abdominal thrusts used). If there is any suspicion part of the object is still in the respiratory tract or any intra-abdominal injuries as a result of abdominal thrusts, refer to A&E.

If the child is UNCONSCIOUS: ❶ Don't leave the child
- Place on a firm, flat surface—call out/send for help if not arrived
- Open the mouth and look for any obvious object. If one is seen, make an attempt to remove it with a single finger sweep.
- Open the airways and attempt 5 rescue breaths. Assess effectiveness of each breath—if a breath doesn't make the chest rise, reposition the head before making the next attempt.
- If there is no response to the rescue breaths, proceed immediately to chest compression—regardless of whether the breaths were successful. Follow the PBLS sequence (📖 p.24) for 1 min before summoning help if not already there.

If it appears the obstruction has been relieved: Open and check the airways. Deliver rescue breaths if the child is not breathing. If the child regains consciousness and is breathing effectively, place him in a safe side-lying (recovery) position and monitor breathing and conscious level while awaiting the arrival of the emergency services.

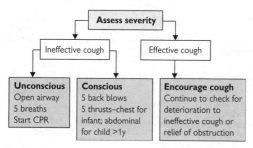

Fig. 5.2 Algorithm for management of paediatric foreign body airway obstruction (PFBAO).

Back blows for small children/infants

- Place the child in a head-downwards, prone position (e.g. across your lap). Support the head if needed by holding the jaw
- Deliver a smart blow with the heel of one hand to the middle of the back between the shoulder blades. Repeat up to 5 times as needed.

Back blows for older children

- Support the child in a forward-leaning position
- Deliver a smart blow with the heel of one hand to the middle of the back between the shoulder blades from behind. Repeat up to 5 times as needed.

Chest thrusts for infants <1 y

- Turn the child into a supine position with head down (e.g. by holding the child's occiput and laying the child along your arm, supported on your thigh)
- Deliver 5 sharp chest thrusts (like chest compressions but slower rate ~20/min) to a point 1 finger's breadth above the xiphisternum.

Abdominal thrusts for children ≥1 y

- Stand behind the child (kneel if small child). Place your arms under the child's arms and encircle his torso
- Clench your fist and place it between the umbilicus and xiphisternum
- Grasp your clenched hand with your other hand and pull sharply inwards and upwards. Repeat up to 5 times as needed.
- ❶ Ensure that pressure is not applied to the xiphoid process or the lower rib cage as this may cause abdominal trauma.

Further information

Resuscitation Council (UK) Resuscitation Guidelines 2005 🖥 www.resus.org.uk

Stridor

Noise created on inspiration due to narrowing of the larynx or trachea. Much more common in children than adults.

⚠ **Signs of severe airways narrowing**
- Distress
- ↑ respiratory rate
- Pallor and cyanosis
- Use of accessory muscles and tracheal tug.

Causes
- Congenital abnormalities of the larynx
- Epiglottis
- Croup (laryngotracheobronchitis)
- Inhaled foreign body
- Trauma
- Laryngeal paralysis.

⚘ **Croup**
- Common viral infection occurring in epidemics in autumn and spring.
- Starts with mild fever and runny nose.
- In younger children (<4 y), oedema and secretions in the larynx and trachea results in a barking cough and inspiratory stridor.
- The cough typically starts at night and is exacerbated by crying and parental anxiety.
- Some children have recurrent attacks associated with viral upper respiratory tract (URTI).

Management
- Steam helps.
- There is also evidence that nebulized steroids can be helpful but most GPs don't carry them.
- Admit as a paediatric emergency if there is intercostal recession, cyanosis or the child's carers are unable to cope.

☼ **Acute epiglottitis**: bacterial infection causing a swollen epiglottis. Potentially, can obstruct the airways. Much rarer since introduction of routine Haemophilus influenza type b (HIB) immunization.

Presentation: look for stridor, drooling, fever, upright leaning forward posture.

⚠ If suspected DON'T examine the child's throat as this can precipitate complete obstruction.

Management
Child: refer as an emergency but try to maintain a calm atmosphere to avoid distressing the child. Examination will be undertaken in hospital with full resuscitation facilities on hand. *Treatment:* IV antibiotics.

Adult: adult epiglottitis is less likely to cause complete airway obstruction but still has a 5–10% mortality. Refer as an emergency for IV antibiotics.

⊜ **Laryngomalacia (congenital laryngeal stridor):** common among small babies. Owing to floppy aryatic folds and the small size of the airways in young children. Stridor becomes more noticeable during sleep, excitement, crying and with concurrent URTIs. Normally resolves without treatment but parental concern may necessitate referral.

⊛ **Inhaled foreign body:** refer as an emergency to ENT for assessment.

Advice for carers of children with croup

Croup can be very frightening for carers of children. Young children often become worse late at night. Carers may not know what to do and can feel helpless.

Explain the natural history of croup: symptoms may worsen for 1–3 d and then tend to improve over the next week.

Give advice on self-management
- *Stay calm.* Reassure the child. Showing anxiety can frighten the child, cause him or her to become upset and cry, which in turn can make breathing more difficult.
- *Sit the child upright.*
- *Keep the child cool*—remove the child's clothes and give paracetamol and/or ibuprofen.
- *Try a steamy environment,* e.g. sit in the bathroom with the door and window closed and the hot tap running (keep child away from the hot water)—alternatively try taking the child outside into the fresh air.

Advise carers to call a doctor/NHS Direct for advice if:
- The child is struggling for breath—difficulty rather than noise is what is important
- The child's breathing becomes more rapid
- The child becomes very restless
- The child is drooling or unable to swallow
- The child's colour changes from pink to being very pale or tinged blue.

❶ A significant number of children end up being admitted to hospital for observation—often only for 24 h.

☼ Acute breathlessness in adults

Attend as soon as possible after receiving the call for help. If there is likely to be any delay, call for emergency ambulance assistance.

On arrival

- Be calm and reassuring.
- Breathlessness is frightening and panic only adds to the sensation of being breathless.
- Direct history and examination to finding the cause as quickly as possible.
- Treat according to the cause.
- If no cause can be found—don't delay—admit to hospital as an acute medical emergency.

Causes: see Table 5.1.

Acute left ventricular failure (acute LVF): severe acute breathlessness due to pulmonary oedema. Urgent action is needed to save life.

Presenting features

- Sudden acute breathlessness
- Fatigue
- Cough ± haemoptysis (usually pink and frothy)
- Tends to occur at night
- Some relief gained from sitting/standing.

Signs

- Dyspnoea
- Tachycardia—gallop rhythm may be present
- Coarse wet sounding crackles at both bases
- Ankle/sacral oedema if right heart failure also present
- ± hypotension.

Action

- If severe call for ambulance support
- Sit the patient up
- Be reassuring—it is very frightening to be very short of breath
- Give 100% oxygen if available and no history of COPD (24% if history of COPD)
- Give IV furosemide 40–80 mg slowly (or bumetanide 1–2 mg)
- Give IV morphine or diamorphine 2.5–5 mg over 5 min
- Give metoclopramide 10 mg IV (can be mixed with diamorphine)
- Give GTN spray 2 puffs sublingually.

Admission: depends on severity and cause of attack, response to treatment and social support. *Always admit if:*

- Alone at home
- Inadequate social support
- Suspected cause of acute LVF warrants admission (e.g. acute MI)
- Very breathless and no improvement over ½ h with treatment at home
- Hypotension or arrythmia.

Table 5.1 Causes of acute breathlessness

Diagnosis	Features
Asthma ⬜ p.90–96	Breathlessness and wheeze. Usually in association with a past history of asthma though can present *de novo*. Signs of a severe attack include: inability to speak in sentences, tachycardia, pulsus paradoxus, ↑ respiratory rate, use of accessory muscles of respiration, drowsiness or exhaustion.
Anaphylaxis ⬜ p.45–47	1 or both of: • Respiratory difficulty, e.g. wheeze, stridor • Hypotension *Other features may include:* erythema, angio-oedema, generalized pruritus or itching of the palate and/or external auditory meatus, rhinitis, nausea ± vomiting, palpitations, urticaria, conjunctivitis, sense of impending doom.
Acute left ventricular failure ⬜ p.78	*Symptoms:* *Signs:* Sudden acute breathlessness Dyspnoea Fatigue Tachycardia ± gallop rhythm Cough ± haemoptysis Coarse crackles at both bases Tends to occur at night Ankle/sacral oedema if right Some relief from heart failure also present sitting/standing ± hypotension
Arrythmia ⬜ p.60–67	Usually palpitations (though not always) associated with chest pain, collapse or funny turns, sweating, breathlessness and/or hyperventilation. May be a PMH/FH of similar symptoms. or thyroid disease.
PE ⬜ p.80	Acute dyspnoea, sharp chest pain (worse on inspiration), haemoptysis and/or syncope. Tachycardic and mild pyrexia.
Acute exacerbation of COPD ⬜ p.88	Worsening of previously stable COPD. Presents with ≥1 of ↑ dyspnoea ↑ cough ↓ exercise tolerance ↑ sputum purulence ↑ fatigue ↑ sputum volume ↑ fluid retention Upper airways symptoms, e.g. cold, ↑ wheeze sore throat Chest tightness New onset cyanosis Acute confusion
Pneumonia ⬜ p.82–85	Breathlessness, cough, fever, sputum, ± sharp, localized chest pain, worse on inspiration.
Pneumothorax ⬜ p.81	Sudden onset of pleuritic chest pain or ↑ breathlessness ± pallor and tachycardia.
Choking ⬜ p.72–75	Think of aspirated foreign bodies in any history of sudden onset of stridor or symptoms of respiratory distress.
SVC obstruction	Acute breathlessness, headache worse on stooping, swelling of the face and/or neck with fixed elevation of JVP—admit for assessment
Air hunger due to shock ⬜ p.48	Inadequate blood flow to the peripheral circulation—usually associated with ↓ BP (± tachycardia) and peripheral cyanosis.
Hyper-ventilation ⬜ p.246	Breathlessness associated with fear, terror and a sense of impending doom

⚙ Pulmonary embolism and pneumothorax

Pulmonary embolism (PE): venous thrombi—usually from a DVT in the leg—pass into the pulmonary circulation and block blood flow to the lungs. Without treatment 20% with proximal DVT develop PE. Fatal in ~1:10 cases causing ~20,000 deaths/y in UK hospitals.

Risk factors
- Immobility: long flight or bus journey, post-op, plaster cast
- Smoking
- COC pill
- Pregnancy or puerperium
- Malignancy
- Past history or family history of DVT or PE.

Presentation
Symptoms: acute dyspnoea, pleuritic chest pain, haemoptysis, syncope. Large clots can be rapidly fatal.

Signs
- Hypotension
- Tachycardia
- Cyanosis
- Tachypnoea
- Pleural rub
- ↑JVP

Look for a source of emboli—though often DVT is not clinically obvious.

⚠ Have a high level of suspicion. Patients may have minimal symptoms/signs apart from some pleuritic pain and dyspnoea. PE in the community can be linked with surgical procedures done 2–3 wk previously.

Differential diagnosis
- Pneumonia and pleurisy
- MI/unstable angina
- Other causes of acute breathlessness—acute LVF, asthma, exacerbation of COPD, pneumothorax, shock (e.g. due to anaphylaxis), arrythmia, hyperventilation
- Other causes of acute chest pain—aortic dissection, rib fracture, musculoskeletal chest pain, pericarditis, oesophageal spasm, shingles.

Immediate action: if suspected, give oxygen as soon as possible and admit as an acute medical emergency.

Further management: in all cases of proven PE, anticoagulation is started in hospital or by a hospital-at-home service before discharge to general practice. Warfarin should be continued for 6 mo. Aim to keep the INR ≈2.5 (range 2–3).

Pneumothorax

Spontaneous pneumothorax—risk factors:
- Previous pneumothorax
- Smoking
- Ascent in an aeroplane
- Diving

Cause
- *In patients <40 y:* usually due to rupture of a pleural bleb. Typical patient is tall, thin and male ($\male:\female \approx 6:1$)
- *Patients >40 y:* usually due to COPD (70–80%)
- *Rarer causes:* asthma, pneumonia, TB, lung cancer, pulmonary fibrosis.

Presentation: sudden onset of pleuritic chest pain or ↑ breathlessness ± pallor and tachycardia. Look for resonant percussion note, ↓ or absent breath sounds—signs may be absent if the pneumothorax is small.

Management
- Refer for CXR
- If pneumothorax is confirmed, seek specialist advice about further management.
- Small pneumothoraces usually resolve spontaneously (50% collapse takes ~40 d to resorb)—monitor until completely resolved.
- Larger pneumothoraces may require admission for aspiration or a chest drain.
- Smoking cessation ↓ risk of recurrence.

Traumatic pneumothorax: trauma may not initially be obvious—ask about injections around the chest area, e.g. acupuncture (to neck and shoulders as well as chest); aspiration of breast lump, etc. Presentation and management is as for spontaneous pneumothorax (above).

Tension pneumothorax: complication of traumatic pneumothorax; rare after spontaneous pneumothorax. A valvular mechanism develops—air is sucked into the pleural space during inspiration but cannot be expelled during expiration. The pressure within the pleural space ↑, the lung deflates further, the mediastinum shifts to the opposite side of the chest and venous return ↓. Can be rapidly fatal.

Clinical features
- Agitated and distressed patient often with a history of chest trauma
- Tachycardia
- Sweating
- Signs of a large pneumothorax: ↓ breath sounds and ↓ chest movement on the affected side
- Mediastinal shift: trachea deviated away from the side of the pneumothorax

Action: If tension pneumothorax is suspected
- Sit the patient upright if possible
- Insert a large bore cannula through the 2nd intercostal space of the chest wall in the mid-clavicular line on the side of the pneumothorax to relieve the pressure in the pleural space
- Transfer as an emergency to hospital.

🔔 Children's respiratory tract infections

Bronchiolitis: occurs in epidemics—usually in the winter months. 70% of infections are due to respiratory syncitial virus (RSV) infection. Usually infects infants of <1 y and presents with coryzal symptoms progressing to irritable cough, rapid breathing ± feeding difficulty.

Children at high risk of severe bronchiolitis: have a low threshold for admission.
• Premature babies
• Babies <6 wk old
• Children with underlying lung disease, e.g. cystic fibrosis
• Children with congenital heart disease
• Immunosuppressed children.

❶ Palivizumab is a monoclonal antibody indicated for the prevention of RSV infection in infants at high risk of infection. Prescribe *only* under specialist supervision and on the basis of likelihood of hospitalization. Give the first dose before the start of the RSV season and then give monthly throughout the RSV season.

Examination: tachypnoea, tachycardia, widespread crepitations over the lung fields ± high pitched wheeze.

Management: depends on severity of the symptoms.
• *If mild*—paracetamol as required and fluids. Bronchodilators may give short-term benefit. There is no evidence antibiotics or steroids help.
• *If more severe*, i.e. if the child or parent is distressed, the child is unable to feed, dehydrated, and/or there is intercostal recession or cyanosis—admit as a paediatric emergency for oxygen ± tube feeding. Rarely ventilation is required.

Prognosis: a proportion of children who have had bronchiolitis as babies, will wheeze with URTIs as small children.

Childhood pneumonia: diagnosis can be difficult in a child as typical signs may not be evident on first presentation. Do listen to the chest again if the child re-presents even shortly after initial assessment. Typical symptoms/signs include all or some of:
• Fever (bacterial cause is likely if <3 y old and fever >38.5°C)
• Malaise
• Anorexia
• Cough ± purulent sputum
• Tachypnoea and/or other signs of respiratory difficulty, e.g. expiratory grunt, chest recession. For older children difficulty breathing is more helpful than clinical signs.
• Tachycardia
• Pleuritic chest pain
• Abdominal pain due to pleural inflammation and/or mesenteric adenitis
• Focal chest signs—coarse crackles, reduced breath sounds, bronchial breathing. Generalized wheeze is often due to viral infection.
❶ Always consider chest infection if the child is ill and there is no other explanation.

Aetiology: community acquired pneumonia may be caused by:
- Viral infection: 14–35%—more common in younger children
- Bacterial infection: 10–30%—more common in older children.
  The organism most commonly isolated is *Streptococcus pneumoniae*
  followed by mycoplasma then chlamydia.
- Mixed infection: 8–40%
- No pathogen isolated: 20-60%

Differential diagnosis
- URTI ± transmitted upper airways noise
- Asthma or other wheezing disorder
- Congenital abnormality, e.g. tracheo-oesophageal fistula.

Investigations: often unnecessary in general practice. Consider:
- Pulse oximetry (if available) to assess severity
- CXR—only if diagnostic uncertainty/symptoms are not resolving
- Blood—FBC (↑ WCC); ESR (↑); acute and convalescent titres for
  atypical pneumonia

Management (Table 5.2)
- If symptoms are mild, advise paracetamol and fluids and adopt a watch
  and see approach, or supply with an interval prescription to use if
  symptoms are not resolving after 4–5 d or worsening meanwhile.
- Otherwise, treat with a broad-spectrum antibiotic, e.g. amoxicillin or
  erythromycin (if penicillin allergic or aged >5 y). Advise parents to
  return for GP review if not improving in 48 h or worse in the interim.
- If dehydrated, distressed, not responding to simple antibiotics or any
  complications—admit for paediatric assessment.

Recurrent chest infection: consider further investigation and/or referral
to look for an underlying cause, if a child has a history of ≥2 probable
chest infections.

Upper respiratory tract infection 🕮 p.120

Influenza: 🕮 p.86.

Croup: 🕮 p.76.

Table 5.2 Which children should be admitted to hospital?

Infants (<1 y)	Older children
Oxygen saturation <92%	Oxygen saturation <92%
Cyanosis	Cyanosis
Respiratory rate >70 breaths/min	Respiratory rate >50 breaths/min
Difficulty breathing	Difficulty breathing
Intermittent apnoea	Grunting
Grunting	Signs of dehydration
Not feeding	Family unable to manage
Family unable to manage	Family unable to provide adequate observation/supervision
Family unable to provide adequate observation/supervision	

🔔 Adult pneumonia

Common condition with annual incidence of ~8 cases/1000 adult population. Incidence ↑ with age and peaks in the winter. Mortality for those managed in the community is <1% but 1 in 4 patients with pneumonia are admitted to hospital and mortality for those admitted is ~9%.

Presentation: acute illness characterized by:
- Symptoms of an acute lower respiratory tract illness (cough + ≥1 other lower respiratory tract symptom, e.g. purulent sputum, pleurisy)
- New focal chest signs on examination (consolidation or ↓ air entry, coarse crackles and/or pleural rub)
- ≥1 systemic feature
  - Sweating, fevers, shivers, aches and pains *and/or*
  - Temperature ≥38°C
- No other explanation for the illness.

❶ The elderly may present atypically, e.g. 'off legs' or acute confusion.

Investigations: often unnecessary in general practice. Consider:
- *Pulse oximetry* (if available): use to assess severity. If oxygen saturation ≤92% in air, the patient is hypoxic and requires admission.
- *CXR:* if diagnostic uncertainty or symptoms not resolving. CXR changes may lag behind clinical signs but should return to normal <6 wk after recovery. Persistent changes on CXR >6 wk after recovery require further investigation.
- *Sputum culture:* if not responding to treatment. If weight ↓, malaise, night sweats or risk factors for TB (ethnic origin, history of TB exposure, social deprivation or elderly) request mycobacterium culture.
- *Blood:* FBC: ↑ WCC; ESR ↑; acute and convalescent titres to confirm 'atypical' pneumonia (Legionella, *C. psittaci, M. pneumonia*).

Differential diagnosis
- Pneumonitis, e.g. 2° to radiotherapy, chemical inhalation
- Pulmonary oedema (may co-exist in the elderly)
- PE
- Acute bronchitis
- Exacerbation of COPD
- Lung cancer
- Bronchiectasis.

Management
Consider the need for admission: Figure 5.3.
- Have a low threshold for admission if
  - ill but apyrexial
  - concomitant illness (e.g. CCF, chronic lung, renal or liver disease, DM, cancer) *or*
  - poor social situation.
- If life-threatening infection or considerable delay (>2 h) before admission, consider administering antibiotics before admission.

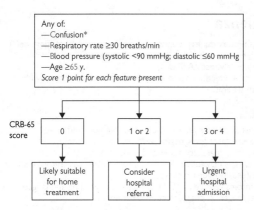

Any of:
—Confusion*
—Respiratory rate ≥30 breaths/min
—Blood pressure (systolic <90 mmHg; diastolic ≤60 mmHg
—Age ≥65 y.
Score 1 point for each feature present

| CRB-65 score | 0 | 1 or 2 | 3 or 4 |

| Likely suitable for home treatment | Consider hospital referral | Urgent hospital admission |

*Defined as a mental test score of ≤8, or new disorientation in person, place or time.

Fig. 5.3 Assessment of severity and management of adult pneumonia.

If a decision is made to treat at home
- Advise not to smoke, to rest and drink plenty of fluids
- Start antibiotics, e.g. amoxicillin 500 mg–1 g tds, erythromycin 500 mg qds or clarithromycin 500 mg bd
- Treat pleuritic pain with simple analgesia, e.g. paracetamol 1 g qds
- Review within 48 h. Reassess clinical state
- If deteriorating or not improving consider CXR or admission.

Possible reasons why patients may not improve
- Elderly—slow clinical response
- Incorrect diagnosis
- Incorrect antibiotics, e.g. antibiotic resistance
- Non-bacterial cause, e.g. viral, fungal
- TB
- Impaired immunity, e.g. HIV
- Secondary complication, e.g. pleural effusion, lung abscess.

⚠ Prevention: *Offer:*
- *Influenza vaccination* to high-risk individuals: ≥65 y, chronic renal, lung, liver or heart disease (excluding ↑ BP alone), DM, immuno-compromised/asplenic patients, patients living in long-term residential care, carers of patients with disabilities, and health professionals.
- *Pneumococcal vaccination* to high-risk individuals: ≥65 y, chronic renal disease or nephrotic syndrome, chronic lung, liver or heart disease, DM, immunocompromised or asplenic patients, coeliac disease, cochlear implant, CSF shunts, children <5 y who have had previous invasive pneumococcal disease and have not been vaccinated as part of the routine vaccination programme.

△ Influenza

Sporadic respiratory illness during autumn and winter causing ≈600 deaths/y with epidemics every 2–3 y → 10× ↑ in deaths.
- *Causes:* influenza viruses A, B or C.
- *Spread:* droplet infection, person-to-person contact, or contact with contaminated items.
- *Incubation:* 1–7 d.

Presentation
- In mild cases symptoms are like those of a common cold.
- In more severe cases fever begins suddenly accompanied by prostration and generalized aches and pains.
- Other symptoms may follow: headache, sore throat, respiratory tract symptoms (usually cough ± coryza).
- Acute symptoms resolve in <5 d but weakness, sweating and fatigue may persist longer. 2° chest infection is common.

Management
- *Symptomatic:* rest, fluids and paracetamol for fever/symptom control.
- *Treatment of secondary complications:* e.g. antibiotics for chest infection, persistent otitis media or tonsillitis/pharyngitis; treatment of exacerbations of COPD or asthma.
- *Antivirals:* Zanamivir (Relenza™ 10 mg bd for 5 d by inhalation) and Oseltamivir (Tamiflu™ 75 mg bd for 5d) are not a 'cure' but may shorten duration of symptoms and ↓ incidence of complications if started <48 h after onset of symptoms. Antivirals should only be used for treatment of patients in high-risk groups (Box 5.2—except in pregnancy) and only when influenza is prevalent in the community[N]. Zanamivir should only be used for adults; Oseltamivir can be used for adults or children >1 y.

⚠ Zanamivir may cause bronchospasm—ensure a short-acting bronchodilator is available if the patient has a tendency to bronchospasm. Avoid in severe asthma unless close monitoring and facilities to treat bronchospasm are available.

Prevention
- Influenza vaccine is prepared each year from viruses of the 3 strains thought most likely to cause 'flu' that winter. It is ~70% effective (range 30–90%). Protection lasts 1 y. Give to high-risk groups—Box 5.2. Practices may give influenza vaccination as a direct enhanced service and points are available via the QOF for vaccination of high-risk patients.
- Oseltamivir is recommended for prophylaxis in high-risk patients >13 y who are not effectively vaccinated or who live in residential care where a staff member has influenza-like symptoms only when influenza is prevalent in the community. Use at a dose of 75 mg od for 7–10 d from diagnosis of the latest case in the establishment[N].

❶ Community-based virological surveillance schemes will indicate when influenza is circulating in the community

Influenza pneumonia: the principal viral cause of pneumonia is influenza A virus. This usually occurs during epidemics of influenza A—Asian 'flu'—but is rare. May affect previously healthy individuals but patients with underlying disease, e.g. COPD are at greater risk. *Features:*
- Develops rapidly
- Presents with progressive dyspnoea
- Acute haemorrhagic disease of the lungs may cause death within hours
- Treatment is supportive and, if detected early enough, with antivirals.

❶ The most common cause of pneumonia during influenza epidemics is secondary bacterial infection, usually with *Staphylococcus aureus* or *Streptococcus pneumoniae*.

Bird flu
- A severe form of avian influenza or 'bird flu'—called H5N1—has affected poultry flocks and other birds in several countries since 2003.
- >150 people have caught the infection, as a result of close and direct contact with infected birds and >½ have subsequently died.
- There is no firm evidence that H5N1 has acquired the ability to pass easily from person to person.
- Concern remains that the virus might develop the ability to pass from person to person, or that it might mix with human flu viruses to create a new virus and create a new human flu pandemic.

Box 5.2

Patients at risk of developing severe disease with influenza:
- aged ≥65 y or
- with ≥ 1 of the following conditions:
  - chronic respiratory disease including COPD and asthma
  - significant cardiovascular disease excluding hypertension
  - chronic renal disease
  - immunosuppression (including hyposplenism)
  - diabetes mellitus.

Indications for influenza vaccination:
- aged ≥65 y
- chronic renal disease
- DM
- chronic liver disease
- chronic lung disease, e.g. asthma, COPD
- cardiovascular disease (except ↑BP alone)
- immunocompromised or asplenic patients
- carers of patients with disabilities
- patients living in long-stay residential care establishments
- health professionals expected to be in contact with influenza.

Further information

NICE Guidance on the use of Zanamivir, Oseltamivir and Amantadine for the treatment of influenza (2003) ▣ www.nice.org.uk
Health Protection Agency (HPA) Topics A-Z: Influenza ▣ www.hpa.org.uk

🔔 Acute exacerbations of COPD

Presentation: worsening of previous stable condition.

Features: ≥1 of
- ↑ dyspnoea—marked dyspnoea, tachypnoea (>25 breaths/min), use of accessory muscles at rest and purse lip breathing are signs of severe exacerbation
- ↓ exercise tolerance—marked ↓ in activities of daily living is a sign of severe exacerbation
- ↑ fatigue
- ↑ fluid retention—new onset oedema is a sign of severe exacerbation
- ↑ wheeze
- Chest tightness
- ↑ cough
- ↑ sputum purulence
- ↑ sputum volume
- Upper airways symptoms, e.g. colds, sore throats
- New onset cyanosis—severe exacerbation
- Acute confusion—severe exacerbation.

❶ Fever and chest pain are uncommon presenting features—consider alternative diagnosis.

Causes of exacerbations: 30% have no identifiable cause.
- *Infections:* viral upper and lower respiratory tract infections, e.g. common cold, influenza; bacterial lower respiratory tract infections.
- *Pollutants,* e.g. nitrous oxide, sulphur dioxide, ozone.

Differential diagnosis

- Pneumonia
- LVF/pulmonary oedema
- Lung cancer
- Pleural effusion
- Recurrent aspiration.
- Pneumothorax
- PE
- Upper airways obstruction

Investigations

- *Pulse oximetry:* if available can be used as a measure of severity (saturation ≤92% breathing air suggests hypoxaemia—consider admission) and to monitor progress.
- *CXR:* consider if diagnostic doubt and/or to exclude other causes of symptoms
- *Sputum culture:* not recommended routinely in the community[G]

Management: decide whether to treat at home or admit to hospital—Table 5.3.

Home treatment of acute exacerbations

- *Add or ↑ bronchodilators.* Consider if inhaler device and technique are appropriate.
- *Start antibiotics:* use broad-spectrum antibiotic, e.g. erythromycin 250–500 mg qds if sputum becomes more purulent *or* clinical signs of pneumonia *or* consolidation on CXR.

- *Oral corticosteroids:* start early in the course of the exacerbation if ↑ breathlessness that interferes with daily activities. Dosage: 30 mg/d of prednisolone for 1–2 wk. Consider osteoporosis prophylaxis with a bisphosphonate if frequent courses are required.

Follow-up
- Reassess as necessary. If the patient deteriorates reconsider the need for hospital admission. If not fully improved in within 2 wk consider CXR and hospital referral.
- Reassess patients who have been admitted 4–6 wk after discharge. Assess their ability to cope at home. ~1:3 are readmitted within 3 mo.
- Reassess inhaler technique and understanding of treatment regimen.
- In severe cases, reassess the need for LTOT and/or home nebulizer.
- Check FEV_1
- Emphasize the potential benefit of lifestyle modification—smoking cessation, exercise, weight loss if obese.
- Arrange ongoing regular follow-up.

Further information
RCP/NICE National clinical guideline on management of chronic obstructive pulmonary disease in adults in primary and secondary care (2004). Thorax 59 (Suppl.1) 1-232.

Table 5.3 Deciding whether to treat acute exacerbations at home or in hospital (the more features in the 'treat in hospital column', the more likely the need for admission)

	Treat at home	Treat in hospital*
Ability to cope at home	Yes	No
Breathlessness	Mild	Severe
General condition	Good	Poor—deteriorating
Level of activity	Good	Poor/confined to bed
Cyanosis	No	Yes
Worsening peripheral oedema	No	Yes
Level of consciousness	Normal	Impaired
Already receiving LTOT	No	Yes
Social circumstances	Good	Living alone/not coping
Acute confusion	No	Yes
Rapid rate of onset	No	Yes
Significant co-morbidity (e.g. cardiac disease, IDDM)	No	Yes
Changes on CXR (if available)	No	Present

* Hospital-at-home schemes and assisted discharge schemes are a suitable alternative.

Reproduced with permission of BMJ journals.

:☼: **Acute asthma in adults**

Many deaths from asthma are preventable. Delay can be fatal. Factors leading to poor outcome include:
- Doctors failing to assess severity by objective measurement
- Patients or relatives failing to appreciate severity
- Underuse of corticosteroids

⚠ Regard each emergency asthma consultation as acute severe asthma until proven otherwise

Risk factors for developing fatal or near fatal asthma
A combination of severe asthma recognized by ≥1 of:
- Previous near fatal asthma (see opposite)
- Previous admission for asthma—especially if within 1 y
- Requiring ≥3 classes of asthma medication
- Heavy use of β_2 agonist
- Repeated attendances at A&E for asthma care—especially if within 1 y
- Brittle asthma.

and adverse behavioural or psychosocial features recognized by ≥1 of:
- Non-compliance with treatment or monitoring
- Failure to attend appointments
- Self-discharge from hospital
- Psychosis, depression, other psychiatric illness or deliberate self-harm
- Current or recent major tranquillizer use
- Denial
- Alcohol or drug misuse
- Obesity
- Learning difficulties
- Employment/income problems
- Social isolation
- Childhood abuse
- Severe marital/legal/domestic stress

Assess and record
- Peak expiratory flow (PEF)
- Symptoms and response to self-treatment
- Heart and respiratory rates
- Oxygen saturation by pulse oximetry (if available)

⚠ Patients with severe or life-threatening attacks may not be distressed and may not have all the characteristic abnormalities of severe asthma. The presence of any should alert the doctor

Levels of severity of acute asthma exacerbations
Moderate asthma exacerbation
- Increasing symptoms
- PEF >50–75% predicted
- No features of acute severe asthma

Acute severe asthma: any one of:
- PEF 33–50% best or predicted
- Respiratory rate ≥25 breaths/min

- Heart rate ≥110/min
- Inability to complete sentences in 1 breath

Life-threatening asthma: any 1 of the following with severe asthma:
- PEF <33% best/predicted
- O$_2$ saturation <92%
- Silent chest
- Cyanosis
- Feeble respiratory effort
- Bradycardia
- Dysrhythmia
- Hypotension
- Exhaustion
- Confusion
- Coma

Near fatal asthma: respiratory acidosis and/or requiring mechanical ventilation with ↑ inflation pressures.

Brittle asthma
- *Type 1:* wide PEF variability (>40% diurnal variation for >50% of the time for a period of >150 d) despite intense therapy
- *Type 2:* sudden severe attacks on a background of apparently well-controlled asthma.

Management: Figure 5.4, 📖 p.92.

Admit to hospital if:
- Life-threatening features
- Features of acute severe asthma present after initial treatment
- Previous near fatal asthma

Lower threshold for admission if:
- Afternoon or evening attack
- Recent nocturnal symptoms or hospital admission
- Previous severe attacks
- Patient unable to assess own condition
- Concern over social circumstances

If admitting the patient to hospital:
- Stay with the patient until the ambulance arrives
- Send written assessment and referral details to the hospital
- Give high-dose β$_2$ bronchodilator via an oxygen-driven nebulizer in the ambulance.

Follow-up after treatment or discharge from hospital
- GP review within 48 h
- Monitor symptoms and PEFR
- Check inhaler technique
- Written asthma action plan
- Modify treatment according to guidelines for chronic persistent asthma
- Address potentially preventable contributors to admission.

Further information
BTS/SIGN British guideline on the management of asthma (2004) 🖥 www.sign.ac.uk

Moderate asthma	Acute severe asthma	Life-threatening asthma
INITIAL ASSESSMENT		
PEF>50% best or predicted	PEF 33–50% best or predicted	PEF<33% best or predicted
FURTHER ASSESSMENT		
Speech normal Respiration <25 breaths/min Pulse <110 beats/min	Can't complete sentences Respiration ≥25 breaths/min Pulse ≥110 beats/min	Oxygen saturation <92% Silent chest, cyanosis or feeble respiratory effort Bradycardia, dysrhythmia or hypotension Exhaustion, confusion or coma
MANAGEMENT		
Treat at home or in the surgery and ASSESS RESPONSE TO TREATMENT	Consider admission	Arrange immediate admission
TREATMENT		
High dose β₂ bronchodilator: Ideally via oxygen-driven nebuliser (salbutamol 5 mg or terbutaline 10 mg). Or via a spacer (4–6puffs [given one at a time and inhaled separately] repeated at intervals of 10–20 minutes or air driven nebuliser *If PEF >50–75% predicted/ best:* Give prednisolone 40–50 mg Continue or step up usual treatment *If good response to first nebulized treatment* (symptoms improved, respiration and pulse setting and PEF >50%) – continue or step up usual treatment and continue prednisolone	*Oxygen 40–60% if available* *High dose β₂ bronchodilator:* Ideally via oxygen-driven nebulizer (salbutamol 5 mg or terbutaline 10 mg). Or via a spacer (4–6 puffs [given one at a time and inhaled separately] repeated at intervals of 10–20 minutes *Prednisolone 40–50 mg or IV hydrocortisone 100 mg* *If no response in acute, severe asthma:* ADMIT	*Oxygen 40–60% if available* *Prednisolone 40–50 mg or IV hydrocortisone 100 mg immediately* *High dose β₂ bronchodilator:* and ipratropium Ideally via oxygen-driven nebuliser (salbutamol 5 mg/terbutaline 10 mg) and ipratropium 0.5 mg Or via a spacer (4–6 puffs [given one at a time inhaled separately] repeated at intervals of 10–20 minutes) *ADMIT immediately*

Fig. 5.4 Management of acute severe asthma in adults.

⚙ Acute asthma in children

Assess and record
- Pulse rate—increasing heart rate generally reflects ↑ severity
- Respiratory rate and breathlessness
- Use of accessory muscles—best noted by palpation of neck muscles
- Amount of wheezing
- Degree of agitation and conscious level

Levels of severity
Child >5 y: Figure 5.5.

Child 2–5 y: Figure 5.6, 📖 p.96.

Child <2 y: assessment of children <2 y can be difficult.
- *Moderate wheezing:*
  - O_2 saturation ≥92%
  - Audible wheezing
  - Using accessory muscles
  - Still feeding
- *Severe wheezing:*
  - O_2 saturation <92%
  - Cyanosis
  - Marked respiratory distress
  - Too breathless to feed
- *Life threatening:*
  - Apnoea
  - Bradycardia
  - Poor respiratory effort

⚠ If a patient has signs and symptoms across categories, always treat according to the most severe features

Management
Child >5 y: Figure 5.5.

Child 2–5 y: Figure 5.6, 📖 p.96.

Child <2 y: intermittent wheezing attacks are usually in response to viral infection and response to bronchodilators is inconsistent.
- If mild/moderate wheeze:
  - A trial of bronchodilators can be considered if symptoms are of concern—use a metered dose inhaler and spacer with a face mask.
  - If no response consider alternative diagnosis (aspiration pneumonitis, pneumonia, bronchiolitis, tracheomalacia, CF, congenital anomaly) and/or admit.
- *If severe wheezing:* admit to hospital.
- *If any life-threatening features:* admit immediately as a blue light emergency.

Follow-up after treatment or discharge from hospital
- GP review within 1 wk
- Monitor symptoms, PEFR and check inhaler technique
- Written asthma action plan
- Modify treatment according to guidelines for chronic persistent asthma
- Address potentially preventable contributors to admission.

ASSESS ASTHMA SEVERITY		
Moderate exacerbation	Severe exacerbation	Life threatening asthma
Oxygen saturation ≥92% PEF ≥50% best or predicted Able to talk Heart rate ≤120/min Respiratory rate ≤30/min	Oxygen saturation <92% PEF <50% best or predicted Too breathless to talk Heart rate >120/min Respiratory rate >30/min Use of accessory neck muscles	Oxygen saturation <92% PEF <33% best or predicted Silent chest Poor respiratory effort Agitation Altered consciousness Cyanosis
β_2 agonist 2–4 puffs via spacer Consider soluble prednisolone 30–40 mg	Oxygen via face mask 4–6 puffs of β_2 agonist [given one at a time and inhaled separately] repeated at intervals of 10–20 minutes or nebulised salbutamol 2.5–5 mg or terbutaline 5–10 mg	Oxygen via face mask Nebulize: • salbutamol 5 mg or terbutaline 10 mg + • ipratropium 0.25 mg
Increase β_2 agonist dose by 2 puffs every 2 min up to 10 puffs according to response	Assess response to treatment 15 min after β_2 agonist	Soluble prednisolone 30–40 mg or IV hydrocortisone 100 mg
IF POOR RESPONSE ARRANGE ADMISSION	IF POOR RESPONSE REPEAT β_2 AGONIST AND ARRANGE ADMISSION	REPEAT β_2 AGONIST VIA OXYGEN-DRIVEN NEBULIZER WHILST ARRANGING IMMEDIATE HOSPITAL ADMISSION

GOOD RESPONSE Continue up to 10 puffs or nebulised β_2 agonist as needed (max. every 4 h) If symptoms are not controlled repeat β_2 agonist and refer to hospital Continue prednisolone for up to 3 d Arrange follow up clinic visit	POOR RESPONSE Stay with the patient until the ambulance arrives Send written assessment and referral details Repeat β_2 agonist via oxygen driven nebuliser in the ambulance

⚠ **Lower threshold for admission if**

• Attack in late afternoon or at night
• Recent hospital admission or previous severe attack
• Concern over social circumstances or ability to cope at home.

Fig. 5.5 Management of acute asthma in children >5 y.

ASSESS ASTHMA SEVERITY		
Moderate exacerbation	Severe exacerbation	Life threatening asthma
Oxygen saturation ≥92% Able to talk Heart rate ≤130/min Respiratory rate ≤50/min	Oxygen saturation <92% Too breathless to talk Heart rate >130/min Respiratory rate >50/min Use of accessory neck muscles	Oxygen saturation <92% Silent chest Poor respiratory effort Agitation Altered consciousness Cyanosis
β_2 agonist 2–4 puffs via spacer ± face mask Consider soluble prednisolone 20 mg Increase β_2 agonist dose by 2 puffs every 2 minutes up to 10 puffs according to response	Oxygen via face mask 4–6 puffs of β_2 agonist [given one at a time and inhaled separately] repeated at intervals of 10–20 minutes or nebulised salbutamol 2.5 mg or terbutaline 5 mg Soluble prednisolone 20 mg Assess response to treatment 15 min after β_2 agonist	Oxygen via face mask Nebulize: • salbutamol 2.5 mg or terbutaline 5 mg + • ipratropium 0.25 mg Soluble prednisolone 20 mg or IV hydrocortisone 50 mg
IF POOR RESPONSE ARRANGE ADMISSION	IF POOR RESPONSE REPEAT β_2 AGONIST AND ARRANGE ADMISSION	REPEAT β_2 AGONIST VIA OXYGEN-DRIVEN NEBULIZER WHILST ARRANGING IMMEDIATE HOSPITAL ADMISSION

GOOD RESPONSE	POOR RESPONSE
Continue β_2 agonist via spacer or nebuliser as needed but not exceeding 4 hourly. If symptoms are not controlled repeat β_2 agonist and refer to hospital Continue prednisolone for up to 3 days Arrange follow-up clinic visit	Stay with the patient until the ambulance arrives Send written assessment and referral details Repeat β_2 agonist via oxygen driven nebuliser in the ambulance

⚠ **Lower threshold for admission if**

• Attack in late afternoon or at night
• Recent hospital admission or previous severe attack
Concern over social circumstances or ability to cope at home.

Fig. 5.6 Management of acute asthma in children 2–5 y.

Further information

BTS/SIGN British guideline on the management of asthma (2004) 🖥 www.sign.ac.uk

Figure 5.6 is reproduced from the British guideline on the management of asthma (2004) with permission from SIGN/British Thoracic Society.

Gastrointestinal and urological emergencies

☼ **Acute abdominal pain**

❶ Signs may be masked in elderly patients or those on corticosteroids. Small children with abdominal pain are difficult to assess.

History: consider:
- Site of pain—see Figure 6.1
- Onset: How long? How did it start? Change over time?
- Character of pain: Type of pain—burning, shooting, stabbing, dull, etc.
- Radiation
- Associated symptoms, e.g. nausea, vomiting, diarrhoea
- Timing/pattern e.g. constant, colicky, relationship to food
- Exacerbating and relieving factors
- Severity
- Previous treatments tried and result.

Examination

• Temperature	• Anaemia
• Pulse	• Site of pain (Figure 6.1)
• BP	• Guarding/rebound tenderness
• Jaundice	• Rectal/vaginal examination as necessary

Management: treat the cause (Table 6.1)—if unsure admit as a surgical emergency to hospital. Do not give analgesia prior to surgical assessment as it may mask vital diagnostic signs.

Acute appendicitis: commonest surgical emergency in the UK—lifetime incidence ≈6%. *Peak age:* 10–30 y.

Presentation: central abdominal colic progresses and localizes in the RIF, becoming worse on movement (especially coughing, laughing); anorexia; dysuria; nausea ± vomiting; rarely diarrhoea.

Examination
- Discomfort on walking (tend to walk stooped) and coughing
- Flushed and unwell—pyrexia (~37.5°C)
- Furred tongue and/or foetor oris
- Tenderness and guarding in the right iliac fossa (especially over McBurney's point—$^2/_3$ of the distance between the umbilicus and anterior superior iliac spine) and pain in the right iliac fossa on palpation of the left iliac fossa (Rovsing's sign)
- Rectal/vaginal examination—tender high on the right. No cervical excitation.

Investigation: urinalysis—NAD or trace of blood.

Management: admit as a surgical emergency—expect to be wrong ~½ the time.

⚠ Symptoms and signs may be atypical—especially in the very old/very young. In pregnancy, pain is typically higher. If unsure of diagnosis and the patient is unwell—admit. If well, either arrange to review a few hours later or ask the patient/carer to contact you if any deterioration or change in symptoms occurs.

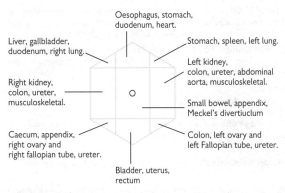

Fig. 6.1 Site of abdominal pain gives important clues about the organ involved.

Table 6.1 Differential diagnosis of acute abdominal pain

Renal and gynaecological causes	GI causes	Other causes
Renal colic— 📖 p.110	Irritable bowel syndrome	Shingles/post-herpetic neuralgia
UTI 📖 p.111	Constipation	Spinal arthritis
Pyelonephritis	Diverticular disease 📖 p.105	Muscular pain
Hydronephrosis	Gallbladder disease—biliary colic, cholecystitis— 📖 p.102	CCF
Henoch–Schoenlein purpura	Liver disease	Sickle cell crisis— 📖 p.264
Ectopic pregnancy— 📖 p.188	Crohn's— 📖 p.106	Ruptured spleen— 📖 p.102
Dysmenorrhoea	UC— 📖 p.106	Torsion of the testis— 📖 p.113
Endometriosis	Gastroenteritis— 📖 p.108	Leaking/ruptured AAA— 📖 p.52
Pelvic inflammatory disease— 📖 p.182	Gastritis	Mesenteric artery ischaemia 📖 p.104
Ovarian torsion	Peptic ulcer	Mesenteric adenitis 📖 p.102
Ovarian cyst— bleed/rupture	Perforated bowel— 📖 p.105	MI— 📖 p.58
Gynaecological malignancy	Appendicitis— 📖 p.100	Pneumonia— 📖 p.84
	Meckel's diverticulum	Subphrenic abscess
	Pancreatitis— 📖 p.103	DM—ketoacidosis— 📖 p.178
	Bowel obstruction— 📖 p.103	Porphyria— 📖 p.265
	Intussusception— 📖 p.104	Addison's— 📖 p.179
	Strangulated hernia— 📖 p.104	Lead poisoning
	Volvulus— 📖 p.103	
	GI malignancy	

Mesenteric adenitis: pain due to mesenteric lymphadenopathy in children. Usually associated with URTI. Treat with simple analgesia and fluids. Review if the pain becomes more severe or changes.

Ruptured spleen: may occur immediately following trauma or present days/weeks later. Diseased spleens (e.g. glandular fever, malaria, leukaemia) rupture more easily.

Presentation
• History of abdominal trauma
• Blood loss: tachycardia, ↓ BP ± postural drop, pallor
• Peritoneal irritation: guarding, abdominal rigidity, shoulder tip pain
• Paralytic ileus: abdominal distention, lack of bowel sounds.

⚠ *Action:* If suspected, admit as a blue-light surgical emergency

Biliary colic: clear-cut attacks of severe upper abdominal pain that may radiate → back/shoulder tip, lasting ≥½ h and causing restlessness ± jaundice ± nausea or vomiting.

Examination: tenderness ± guarding in the right upper quadrant (↑ on deep inspiration—Murphy's sign).

Acute management: treat with pethidine (50 mg IM/po) or diclofenac (50–100 mg IM/po/pr) + prochlorperazine 12.5 mg IM or domperidone 10 mg po/pr for nausea.

Admit as a surgical emergency if:
• Uncertain of diagnosis
• Inadequate social support
• Persistent symptoms despite analgesia
• Suspicion of complications (gallstone ileus, pancreatitis), and/or
• Concomitant medical problems (e.g. dehydration, pregnant, DM, Addison's).

Follow-up: investigate for gallstones with abdominal USS to prove diagnosis when the episode has settled.

Acute cholecystitis: pain and tenderness in the right upper quadrant/epigastrium ± vomiting.

Examination: tenderness ± guarding in the right upper quadrant ± fever ± jaundice.

Acute management: treat with a broad-spectrum antibiotic (e.g. ciprofloxacin) and analgesia as for biliary colic.

Admit as a surgical emergency if:
• Generalized peritonism or very toxic
• Diagnosis uncertain
• Concomitant medical problems (e.g. dehydration, DM, Addison's, pregnancy)
• Inadequate social support, or
• Not responding to medication

Follow-up: as for biliary colic.

Acute pancreatitis: poorly localized, continuous, boring epigastric pain that ↑ over ~1 h—often worse lying down ± radiation to the back (50%). Accompanied by nausea ± vomiting. Most episodes are mild and self limiting but 1:5 patients have a severe attack. Overall mortality ≈5–10%. May be recurrent.

Examination: tachycardia; fever; shock; jaundice; localized epigastric tenderness or generalized abdominal tenderness; abdominal distension ± ↓ bowel sounds; evidence of retroperitoneal haemorrhage (periumbilical and flank bruising—rare).

Management: admit as an acute surgical emergency.

Complications: delayed complications may present in general practice—suspect if persistent pain or failure to regain weight or appetite. Complications include pancreatic necrosis; pseudocyst (localized collection of pancreatic secretions); fistula/abscess formation; bleeding/thrombosis.

Prevention of further attacks
- Avoid factors that may have caused pancreatitis, e.g. alcohol, drugs
- Advise patients to follow a low fat diet
- Treat reversible causes, e.g. hyperlipidaemia, gallstones.

Intestinal obstruction: blockage of the bowel due to either mechanical obstruction or failure of peristalsis (ileus). *Causes:*
- *Obstruction from outside the bowel:* adhesions or bands; volvulus; neighbouring malignancy (e.g. bladder, ovary); obstructed hernia.
- *Obstruction from within the bowel wall:* tumour; infarction; congenital atresia; Hirschsprung's disease; inflammatory bowel disease; diverticulitis.
- *Obstruction in the lumen:* impacted faeces/constipation; bolus obstruction (e.g. swallowed foreign body); gallstone ileus; intussusception; large polyps.
- *Ileus/functional obstruction:* post-op; electrolyte disturbance; uraemia; DM; back pain; anticholinergic drugs.

Presentation: anorexia; nausea; vomiting (may be faeculent) gives relief; colicky central abdominal pain + distension; absolute constipation for stool and gas (if high obstruction constipation may not be absolute).

Examination: uncomfortable and restless; abdominal distension ± tenderness (though no guarding/rebound); active tinkling bowel sounds or quiet/absent bowel sounds (later).

Management: admit as surgical emergency.

Sigmoid volvulus: occurs in people who have redundant colon on a long mesentery with a narrow base. The sigmoid loop twists causing intestinal obstruction. The loop may become ischaemic. *Risk factors:* constipation, laxatives, tranquillizers.

Presentation: acute onset of abdominal distension and colicky abdominal pain with complete constipation and absence of flatus. There may be a history of repeated attacks.

Management: admit acutely to hospital. Treatment is release by passing a flatus tube and/or surgery.

Follow-up: once the condition has been treated, ↓ recurrences by preventing constipation and stopping tranquillizers if possible.

Intussusception: the invagination of one part of the bowel into the lumen of the immediately adjoining bowel. It is the commonest cause of intestinal obstruction in young children (2:1000) and usually occurs in previously healthy children. *Peak age:* 5–18 mo, ♂:♀ ≈2:1.

Presentation: very variable. Always have a high index of suspicion.
- *Abdominal colic*—paroxysms of pain during which the child draws up his legs—the child often screams with the pain and becomes pale. Episodes usually are 10–15 min apart and last 2–3 min but become more frequent with time.
- *Vomiting*—early symptom.
- *Rectal bleeding*—passage of blood ('redcurrent jelly stool') or slime per rectum is a late sign.
- *Sausage-shaped mass in the abdomen*—usually in the right upper quadrant—though not always present.

⚠ The child becomes rapidly worse if not treated early, becoming toxic and developing an obstructive picture with distended abdomen ± faeculent vomiting.

Differential diagnosis: other causes of bowel obstruction; gastroenteritis; constipation; haemolytic uraemic syndrome

Management: admit as an acute surgical emergency. Untreated intussusception is usually fatal.

Irreducible hernia
- Most types of hernia may become irreducible.
- It may be the 1st presentation of a hernia or a complication of a longstanding hernia.
- If obstructed (incarcerated) or strangulated (blood supply to bowel contained within the hernia sac is compromised) the hernia is tender and there are symptoms/signs of small bowel obstruction.

⚠ In all cases, if you are unable to reduce a hernia, admit urgently for surgical assessment.

Ischaemic bowel: interruption of the blood supply of the bowel.
- 1° *ischaemia:* usually due to either mesenteric embolus from the right side of the heart, or venous thrombosis and typically occurs in elderly patients who might have pre-existing heart or vascular disease.
- 2° *ischaemia:* usually due to intestinal obstruction (e.g. strangulated hernia, volvulus, intussusception).

Presentation: sudden onset of abdominal pain that rapidly becomes severe. There may be a history of pain worse after meals prior to this event (mesenteric angina).

Examination: very unwell; shocked; may be in AF; generalized tenderness but normally no guarding/rebound. Often signs are out of proportion to symptoms.

Management: give opiate analgesia. Admit as surgical emergency.

Acute diverticulitis: presents with:
- Altered bowel habit
- Colicky left-sided abdominal pain—may become continuous and cause guarding/peritonism in the left iliac fossa
- Fever
- Malaise ± nausea
- Flatulence.

❶ There may be few abdominal signs in the elderly

Management: treat with oral antibiotics (e.g. co-amoxiclav 375 mg tds, or cefaclor 250–500 mg tds + metronidazole 400 mg tds, or ciprofloxacin 500–750 mg bd). There may also be some benefit from a low residue diet.

Admit as a surgical emergency if:
- Uncertain of diagnosis
- Inadequate social support
- Severe or persistent symptoms despite analgesia
- Suspicion of acute complications.

Complications: diverticular abscess; haemorrhage; perforation; fistula formation; post-infective stricture.

Perforated bowel: the bowel may perforate at any point along its length. Common causes of perforation are peptic ulcers, diverticula, tumours and inflammatory bowel disease.

Perforated peptic ulcer: ill patient, in pain. History of sudden onset epigastric pain ± haematemesis.

Examination: tachycardic, shallow respiration, abdomen tender with guarding ('board-like rigidity') ± absence of dullness to percussion over the liver (if air has escaped into the peritoneal cavity) ± absent bowel sounds.

❶ Posterior gastric ulcers may perforate into the lesser sac, the chemical peritonitis is contained within the lesser sac and symptoms and signs are more insidious.

More distal perforation: ill patient, in pain. History of sudden onset abdominal pain.

Examination: toxic (fever, tachycardia, ↓ BP), abdomen tender with guarding ± absence of dullness to percussion over the liver (if air has escaped into the peritoneal cavity) ± absent bowel sounds.

⚠ In all cases, admit as an acute surgical emergency.

⊛ Acute exacerbations of inflammatory bowel disease

Ulcerative colitis: ulcerative colitis affects the large bowel. Exacerbations of ulcerative colitis may present with diarrhoea (sometimes bloody), and/or abdominal pain. Check for fever, mouth ulcers, tachycardia, abdominal tenderness. Record BP.

Management

⚠ *Admit acutely if:*
- Severe abdominal pain (especially if associated with tenderness)
- Severe diarrhoea (>8×/d) ± bleeding
- Dramatic weight loss
- Fever or other signs of systemic disease.

Treatment of active disease
- Mesalazine 2–4g daily. Topical 5-ASA derivatives are a useful adjunct if troublesome rectal symptoms.
- Add steroids (prednisolone 40 mg od po + rectal preparation) if prompt response is needed or mesalazine is unsuccessful. Review frequently and ↓ dose over 8 wk. Rapid withdrawal ↑ risk of relapse.
- If not responding consider urgent referral to gastroenterology for azathioprine, ciclosporin or infliximab.

Crohn's disease: Crohn's disease may affect any part of the digestive tract and clinical features of exacerbations depend on the site of the disease. Most commonly, exacerbations present with abdominal pain (which may be severe enough to mimic appendicitis), and/or diarrhoea, and/or weight loss. Check for fever, mouth ulcers, tachycardia, abdominal tenderness. Record BP.

Management

⚠ *Admit acutely if:*
- Severe abdominal pain (especially if associated with tenderness)
- Severe diarrhoea (>8×/d) ± bleeding
- Dramatic weight loss
- Bowel obstruction
- Fever >37.5°C, pulse >90 bpm, or other signs of systemic disease.

Management of active ileal and/or colonic disease
- Treat with Mesalazine 4 g daily.
- Add steroids (prednisolone 40 mg od po or budesonide 9 mg daily) if unresponsive to mesalazine. Review frequently and ↓ dose over 8 wk. Avoid use for >3 mo. Rapid withdrawal ↑ risk of relapse.
- Elemental or polymeric diets for 4–6 wk can be a useful adjunct or alternative to steroid treatment—take consultant advice.
- Other medical treatments used with consultant supervision include metronidazole, azathioprine and antitumour necrosis factor (infliximab)
- ❶ For disease elsewhere take specialist advice

Toxic megacolon: life-threatening complication of acute exacerbations of inflammatory bowel disease—typically affecting patients recently diagnosed (60% of cases occur in patients diagnosed <3 y before).

Features
- Systemic toxicity
- Segmental dilatation of the colon to >6 cm diameter

Other symptoms/signs
- Altered consciousness
- Fever
- Tachycardia
- Postural hypotension
- Abdominal tenderness ± localized/generalized peritonitis
- Abdominal distension.

❶ Symptoms/signs may be masked by treatment of an acute exacerbation, e.g. by steroids, analgesics

Management: if suspected, admit as an acute medical emergency.

◉ Vomiting and diarrhoea

History: determine nature and duration of symptoms. If diarrhoea, is there blood/mucus in the stool? If vomiting , colour and frequency; ability to retain food/fluids; nature of vomitus; presence of blood/'coffee grounds'; relationship to eating. Contact with anyone else with similar symptoms? History of recent foreign travel? Other symptoms?

Examination

- *Level of hydration:* BP ± postural drop. Pulse. Sunken eyes, dry tongue, ↓ skin turgor, and sunken fontanelle in babies, are all late signs
- *Abdomen:* masses, distention, tenderness, bowel sounds, hepatomegaly
- *Look for other sources of infection,* e.g. ENT; chest infection; UTI.

Causes of vomiting and diarrhoea in primary care

- *Physiological:* breast-fed babies (loose, often explosive, mustard grain stools), posseting in babies, reflux (usually only vomiting), intermittent loose stools related to diet, irritable bowel syndrome.
- *Gastrointestinal infection:* diarrhoea and/or vomiting. Consider pseudomembranous colitis if recent history of antibiotics. Consider temporary cow's milk intolerance in babies with >2 wk diarrhoea.
- *Other infection:* common cause of vomiting in children, e.g. otitis media, tonsillitis, septicaemia.
- *Acute intra-abdominal disease:* Intussusception (admit), appendicitis (admit), acute obstruction (abdominal distension and vomiting—admit), pyloric stenosis (usually babies <12 wk old—vomiting only, admit).
- *Constipation:* usually overflow of soft stool with soiling ± vomiting.
- *Inflammatory bowel disease or malabsorption*—diarrhoea only.
- *Drugs/toxins,* e.g. opiates (vomiting), diclofenac (diarrhoea).
- *Other cause:* ↑ ICP, head injury, haemolytic uraemic syndrome (consider if child passing blood in stool), anorexia/bulimia, migraine, travel/motion sickness, cerebellar disease, Ménière's disease/labyrinthitis, pregnancy, metabolic (ketoacidosis, uraemia), carcinomatosis.

Management

- *Treat any identified cause.*
- *If diarrhoea, send a stool sample for M,C&S if:* fever, blood in stool, recent return from a tropical climate, immunocompromised, resident in an institution and/or persists >7 d.
- *Rehydration:* encourage clear fluid intake (small amounts frequently) ± rehydration salts (use commercial preparations, e.g. Dioralyte®). Reserve antidiarrhoeals (e.g. loperamide) for patients in whom diarrhoea would be difficult, e.g. immobility, travel, work. ⚠ Never give children antidiarrhoeal agents.
- *Food:* stick to a bland diet avoiding dairy products until diarrhoea has settled. Babies who are breast fed or have not been weaned should continue their normal milk.
- *If dehydrated and unable to replace fluids,* e.g. severe vomiting, child or elderly person refusing to drink—admit.
- *If no cause found and diarrhoea lasts >3 wk or any atypical features* refer for urgent investigation or admit.

Table 6.2 Common causes of gastroenteritis in the UK

Organism/ source	Incubation	Symptoms					Food
		D	V	P	F	O	
Staph. aureus	1–6 h	✓	✓	✓		↓BP	Meat
B. cereus	1–5 h	✓	✓				Rice
C. perfringens	6–24 h	✓		✓			Meat
C. botulinum	12–36 h		✓			Paralysis	Canned food
Salmonella species	12–48 h	✓	✓	✓	✓		Meat, eggs, poultry
Shigella[ND]	48–72 h	✓		✓	✓	Blood in stool	Any food
Campylobacter	48 h–5 d	✓		✓	✓	Blood in stool	Milk, water
E. coli	12–72 h	✓		✓	✓	Blood in stool	Food, water
Y. enterocolitica	24–36 h	✓		✓	✓		Milk, water
Giardia lamblia	1–4 wk	✓					Water
Crypto-sporidium	4–12 d	✓		✓	✓		Water
Listeria						Flu-like illness, pneumonia	Milk products, pâtés, raw vegetables
V. para-haemolyticus	12–24 h	✓	✓	✓			Fish
Rotavirus	1–7 d	✓	✓		✓	Malaise	Food, water
Small viruses	36–72 h	✓	✓		✓	Malaise	Any food
Entamoeba histolytica	1–4 wk	✓		✓	✓	Blood in stool	Food, water
Mushrooms	15 min–24 h	✓	✓	✓		Fits, coma, renal/liver failure	
Scrombrotoxin	10–60 min	✓				Flushes, erythema	Fish
Heavy metals, e.g. zinc	5 min–2 h		✓	✓			
Red beans	1–3 h	✓	✓				

D = diarrhoea; V=vomiting; P=abdominal pain; F=fever; O=other.
❶ suspected food poisoning is a notifiable disease.

⚫ Urinary tract problems

Acute renal failure (ARF): ↓ in renal function over hours/days. No specific symptoms/signs. ↓ in urine output is common. If creatinine and urea are acutely raised diagnose ARF. Refer all cases immediately to the acute medical team. *Causes:* 80% acute tubular necrosis (renal ischaemia due to acute circulatory compromise); renal tract obstruction (5%); glomerulonephritis.

Haemolytic uraemic syndrome: commonest cause of acute renal failure in children. Usually follows a bout of gastroenteritis and is due to *E. coli* toxin. Occasionally occurs in the absence of diarrhoea.

Characteristic features
- acute renal failure
- anaemia
- thrombocytopenia (may result in skin purpura).

Presentation: have a high index of suspicion in any child with bloody diarrhoea. *Other features include:* dehydration, oliguria (though may be polyuria), proteinuria/haematuria, CNS symptoms—irritability, drowsiness, ataxia, coma, ↑ BP is associated with non-diarrhoeal disease

Management: admit as a paediatric emergency. In all cases specialist management (often including dialysis) is required.

Renal colic
Symptoms
- Severe pain, which is always present but has waves of ↑ severity.
- Usually starts abruptly as flank pain, which then radiates around abdomen to groin as stone progresses down ureter.
- May be referred to the testis/tip of penis in a man, or labia majora in a woman.
- Occasionally frank haematuria.
- May be past history or family history of renal stones.

Signs
- Patient is obviously in pain—usually unable to sit still and keeps shifting position to try to get comfortable (in contrast to peritonitis where patients tend to keep still).
- May be pale and sweaty.
- May be mild tenderness on deep abdominal palpation or loin tenderness though often minimal signs.
- If fever suspect infection.

Differential diagnosis: acute appendicitis; diverticulitis; cholecystitis; obstruction; strangulated hernia; testicular torsion; salpingitis; ovarian torsion; ruptured AAA; pyelonephritis; pethidine addiction.

Immediate investigations: dipstick urine if possible for RBCs. If no RBCs consider alternative diagnosis.

Management: stones usually pass spontaneously.
- Give pain relief (diclofenac 75 mg IM or 100 mg pr)
- ↑ fluid intake—though avoid too much fluid

- Sieve urine to catch stones for analysis
- Consider hospital admission if: fever, oliguria, poor fluid intake, pregnant uncertain diagnosis, lives alone, analgesia ineffective or short-lived, symptoms continuing >24 h.
- If not admitted: monitor/review pain relief; monitor/review for complication investigate further.

Further investigation if not admitted: can wait until the next working day.
- *Urine*—M,C&S; RBCs. Consider checking pH of urine (>7.5—infective stones; <5.5—urate stones), checking 'spot' test for urine cystine, and requesting 24 h collection of urine for creatinine clearance, calcium, phosphate and uric acid secretion.
- *Radiology*—KUB X-ray—90% of renal stones are radio-opaque (only urate and xanthine stones are radio-translucent); IVP; consider USS.
- *Blood*—U&E, creatinine, Ca^{2+}, PO_4^{3-}, alkaline phosphatase, uric acid, albumin.
- *Recovered stones*—send for biochemical analysis.

Follow-up: give general advice on prevention of stones (↑ fluid intake to >3 l/24 h, avoid milk). If investigations show any loss of renal function, renal obstruction or remaining stones—refer to urology. Dependent on composition of stones give dietary advice/refer to dietician.

Urinary tract infection (UTI) in adults: UTI is one of the most common conditions seen in primary care. ♀>>♂. 20% of women at any time have asymptomatic bacteriuria and 20–40% of women will have a UTI in their lifetime. *Infecting organisms:* E. coli (>70%), Proteus sp., Pseudomonas sp., streptococci, staphylococci.

Risk factors
- Prior infection
- DM
- Pregnancy
- Stones
- Dehydration
- GU instrumentation
- Catheterization
- Sexual intercourse
- Diaphragm use
- ↓ oestrogen (menopause)
- Urinary stasis (e.g. obstruction)
- Genitourinary (GU) malformations
- Delayed micturition (e.g. on long journeys)

Presentations
- *Cystitis:* frequency, dysuria, urgency, strangury, low abdominal pain, incontinence of urine, acute retention of urine, cloudy or offensive urine, and/or haematuria.
- *Pyelonephritis:* loin pain, fever, rigors, malaise, vomiting, and/or haematuria.

Initial investigation: if uncomplicated UTI in an otherwise healthy woman, test urine with a leucocyte esterase and nitrate dipstick. If +ve treat for UTI. *Reasons to send MSU for M,C &S:*
- Unresolved infection after antibiotics
- Recurrent UTI
- Uncatheterized man with UTI
- Catheterized man or woman with symptomatic UTI
- Child—□ p.118
- Pregnant woman
- Suspected pyelonephritis
- Haematuria—microscopic or macroscopic—always investigate further

Further investigation: consider further investigation with blood tests (U&E, Cr, and/or PSA if >40 y and ♂) and/or radiology (renal tract USS, KUB, IVP) if:

- UTI in a man
- UTI in a child (📖 p.118)
- Recurrent UTI in a woman
- Pyelonephritis
- Unclear diagnosis (e.g. persisting symptoms but negative MSU)
- Unusual infecting organism

Management

Children: 📖 p.118.

Catheterized patients: 90% develop bacteriuria <4 wk after insertion of a catheter. Always confirm suspected UTI with MSU—only treat if symptomatic or *Proteus* species grown. May prove difficult to eliminate. No good evidence bladder instillations help.

Pregnant women: both untreated bacteriuria and frank UTI are associated with preterm delivery and intrauterine growth restriction. Treat for at least 1 wk with suitable antibiotic, e.g. cefalexin 250 mg tds. Check MSU following treatment to ensure infection has cleared.

All other patients
- ↑fluid intake (>3 l/24 h).
- *Alkalinize urine* (e.g. potassium citrate solution) to ease symptoms.
- *Oral antibiotics:* trimethoprim 200 mg bd is a good first choice—80% organisms are sensitive. Use a 3 d course for women with uncomplicated UTI. Use a 2 wk course for men, patients with GU malformations or immunosuppression, relapse (same organism) or recurrent UTI (different organism). Use a 14 d course of a quinolone (e.g. ciprofloxacin 250–500 mg bd) for patents with pyelonephritis.
- *Admission to hospital:* rarely required if dehydrated or extremely systemically unwell.
- *Referral to urology:* if any abnormalities are detected on further investigation or unable to resolve symptoms.

Prostatitis: consider acute prostatitis in all men presenting with symptoms of UTI. Treat with 4 wk course of oral antibiotic that penetrates prostatic tissue, e.g. trimethoprim 200 mg bd.

Acute retention of urine: sudden inability to pass urine → lower abdominal discomfort with inability to keep still. Differentiate from other causes of anuria. ♂ >>♀. *Risk factors:* age >70 y, symptoms of prostatism or poor urinary stream.

Causes

- ♂: prostatic obstruction (82%). Precipitated by constipation, alcohol, drugs (anticholinergics, diuretics), UTI, operation (e.g. day case hernia repair).
- ♀: gynaecological pathology—ovarian cancer, fibromas, prolapse.
- *Rarer causes:* urethral stricture, clot retention, spinal cord compression, bladder stone.

Examination

- Abdomen—palpable bladder
- Rectal examination—enlarged ± irregular prostate
- Perineal sensation.

Investigation: only if catheterizing in the community—catheter specimen of urine to exclude infection. Blood for U&E, Cr, and eGFR.

Management: catheterize (record initial volume drained) *or* refer to urology for catheterization—local policies vary. Treat infection. Refer to District nurse for instruction on management of the catheter. Refer to urology for further assessment and treatment.

Torsion of the testis: peak age 15–30 y.

Presentation: sudden onset severe scrotal pain. May be associate with right iliac fossa pain, nausea and vomiting. *Examination:* tender, hard testis riding higher than the contralateral testis.

Action: admit as an emergency to surgical/urology team.

Epididymo-orchitis: inflammation of the testis and epididymis due to infection. The commonest viral cause is mumps. The commonest bacterial infections are gonococci and coliforms. May occur at any age.

Presentation: acute onset pain in testis; swelling and tenderness of testis/ epididymis; fever ± rigors; may be dysuria and ↑ frequency.

Management: may be difficult to distinguish from torsion of the testis. If in doubt admit for urology/surgical opinion.

Priapism: persistent painful erection not related to sexual desire.

Cause: intracavernosal injection for impotence, idiopathic, leukaemia, sickle cell disease or pelvic tumour.

Treatment: ask the patient to climb stairs (arterial 'steal' phenomenon), apply ice packs. If unsuccessful refer to A&E for aspiration of corpora. Rarely surgery is needed.

Paraphimosis: foreskin is retracted then (due to oedema) unable to be replaced. Commonly occurs in catheterized patients when the catheter is changed.

Management: try to replace foreskin using ice packs (↓ swelling) and lubrication (e.g. KY jelly). If unable to replace the foreskin, admit for surgery.

Balanitis: acute inflammation of glans and foreskin. Common organisms— candida (most common), staphylococci., streptococci., coliforms. Can occur at any age. Commonest in young boys when associated with non-retractile foreskin/phimosis. In elderly patients consider DM.

Management: fungal balanitis responds to topical antifungals, e.g. clotri- mazole cream. Bacterial balanitis responds to oral antibiotics, e.g. fluclox- acillin 250 mg qds. If recurrent or due to phimosis consider referral for circumcision.

Trauma to the foreskin: torn frenulum—seen after poorly lubricated intercourse or if caught in a zip. No treatment required. If recurrent, consider referral for circumcision.

Sick children

⌂ Sick children

Normal respiratory rate in children

- *Neonate*: 30–60 breaths/min
- *Infant*: 20–40 breaths/min
- *1–3 y*: 20–30 breaths/min
- *4–10 y*: 15–25 breaths/min
- *>10 y*: 15–20 breaths/min

❶ Be concerned if respiratory rate >70 breaths/min in children <1 y or >50 breaths/min in older children.

Normal pulse rate in children

- *≤1 y*: **110–160 beats/min**
- *2–5 y*: **95–140 beats/min**
- *5–12 y*: **80–120 beats/min**
- *>12 y*: **60–100 beats/min**

Pyrexia: ↑ temperature – oral >37.5°C; rectal >38°C; axillary >37.3°C; ear >38°C. NICE suggests a traffic light system for assessment: – Table 7.1.

Causes of pyrexia: Childhood infections are the most common cause of fever amongst children in general practice – see 📖 p.118–21. Other causes may present as prolonged fever. Consider cancer (lymphoma; leukaemia); immunological causes (connective tissue/autoimmune disease; sarcoidosis; Kawasaki disease); drugs (e.g. antibiotics); liver/renal disease.

Febrile convulsions: 📖 p.138.

Table 7.1 Traffic light system for assessment of children with fever

Red	Amber	Green
Immediate assessment if life threatening features – in all cases see in <2 h	*See the child the same day. Urgency depends on symptoms/signs reported*	*Give advice on management at home and when to seek further help*
Symptoms/Signs:		
• appears ill	• pallor	• normal colour of skin/lips/tongue
• ↓ consciousness/unresponsiveness	• ↓ response to social cues/excessive drowsiness	• responds normally
• colour – mottled/ashen/blue	• ↓ activity/no smile	• not excessively drowsy
• weak, high-pitched or continuous cry	• nasal flaring	• normal cry/smiles/content
• respiratory rate >60	• ↑ respiratory rate (>50 – aged <6mo; >40 aged >6mo)	• moist mucus membranes
• moderate/severe chest indrawing	• oxygen saturation ≤95% in air	• none of the amber/red symptoms or signs
• ↓ skin turgor	• dry mucous membranes	
• non-blanching rash	• poor feeding in infants	
• bulging fontanelle	• capillary return ≥ 3 seconds	
• neck stiffness	• ↓ urine output	
• status epilepticus	• fever for ≥5 d	
• focal neurological signs/seizures	• swelling of a limb/joint	
• bile stained vomiting	• non-weight bearing/not using an extremity	
• high temperature (0–3 mo >38°C; >3mo >39°C)	• new lump >2 cm	

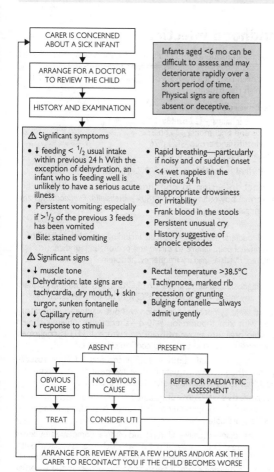

CARER IS CONCERNED
ABOUT A SICK INFANT

↓

ARRANGE FOR A DOCTOR
TO REVIEW THE CHILD

↓

HISTORY AND EXAMINATION

Infants aged <6 mo can be
difficult to assess and may
deteriorate rapidly over a
short period of time.
Physical signs are often
absent or deceptive.

⚠ Significant symptoms

- ↓ feeding < ¹/₂ usual intake
  within previous 24 h With the
  exception of dehydration, an
  infant who is feeding well is
  unlikely to have a serious acute
  illness
- Persistent vomiting: especially
  if >¹/₂ of the previous 3 feeds
  has been vomited
- Bile: stained vomiting

- Rapid breathing—particularly
  if noisy and of sudden onset
- <4 wet nappies in the
  previous 24 h
- Inappropriate drowsiness
  or irritability
- Frank blood in the stools
- Persistent unusual cry
- History suggestive of
  apnoeic episodes

⚠ Significant signs

- ↓ muscle tone
- Dehydration: late signs are
  tachycardia, dry mouth, ↓ skin
  turgor, sunken fontanelle
- ↓ Capillary return
- ↓ response to stimuli

- Rectal temperature >38.5°C
- Tachypnoea, marked rib
  recession or grunting
- Bulging fontanelle—always
  admit urgently

ABSENT   PRESENT

OBVIOUS   NO OBVIOUS   REFER FOR PAEDIATRIC
CAUSE   CAUSE   ASSESSMENT

↓   ↓

TREAT   CONSIDER UTI

ARRANGE FOR REVIEW AFTER A FEW HOURS *AND/OR* ASK THE
CARER TO RECONTACT YOU IF THE CHILD BECOMES WORSE

Arrange for a sick baby not responding to simple measures (e.g. paracetamol
and fluids) to be reviewed by a doctor.

- Trust the mother's instinct.
- Perform a full physical examination. Localizing signs might be absent
  (e.g. tonsillitis can cause vomiting). Petechial rash under the nappy area can
  be easily missed.
- The younger the baby—the lower the threshold for seeking a
  paediatrician's opinion.

Fig. 7.1 General rules for assessment of sick infants.

👁 Childhood infection

There are peaks in incidence of childhood infection when children start nursery, and start and change schools. ❶ Don't forget tropical diseases e.g. malaria in children returning from abroad. Think of TB and endocarditis – especially in high risk patients.

Infections covered elsewhere

- Meningitis/encephalitis – 📖 p.148
- Bronchiolitis and pneumonia – 📖 p.82
- Acute epiglottitis and croup – 📖 p.76
- Diarrhoea and vomiting – 📖 p.108.

Childhood viral infections: Table 7.2, 📖 p.120.

Urinary tract infection in childhood: most childhood UTIs are caused by normal bowel flora—*E. coli* (80%), *Klebsiella*, *Pseudomonas* and other Gram-negative organisms.

Presentation
- *Infants and toddlers:* usually non-specific including vomiting, irritability, fever, abdominal pain, failure to thrive and prolonged jaundice.
- *Older children:* dysuria, urinary frequency, abdominal pain, haematuria, enuresis.

❶ Suspect diagnosis and send urine for M,C&S in any child with urinary symptoms or any infant with fever >38.5°C with no definite cause.

Management: treat symptomatic infection without waiting for laboratory confirmation with trimethoprim for 7–10 d—altering the antibiotic should the responsible organism prove resistant on culture. If UTI is confirmed arrange post-treatment urine testing to confirm clearance.

Follow-up: start prophylactic antibiotics after the first infection (usually trimethoprim od) and continue until further investigations are complete. Refer all children to a paediatrician after the first proven UTI.

Acute suppurative otitis media: caused by viral or bacterial infection, or bacterial infection complicating a viral illness (e.g. URTI, measles)—clinically indistinguishable.

Presentation: ear pain—usually unilateral and often accompanied by fever and systemic upset. There may also be ear discharge associated with relief of pain if there is a spontaneous perforation of the drum. Examination reveals a red, bulging drum. If perforation has occurred the external canal may be filled with pus obscuring the drum. ❶ If you can't see the drum, review the patient after treatment.

Acute management: in 80%, symptoms resolve in ≤3 d without treatment. Advise fluids + paracetamol and/or ibuprofen for analgesia and fever control. Most GPs prescribe antibiotics on presentation (e.g. amoxicillin tds for 5–7 d) if a perforation is present. Otherwise, many GPs use a "delayed" approach—prescribing if symptoms are no better in 3 d.

Prevention: parental smoking ↑ children's risk of otitis media. Encourage patents to stop smoking.

Sore throat: 70% sore throats are viral in origin—the rest bacterial (mostly Group A β-haemolytic streptococci). Viral and bacterial infections are indistinguishable clinically but association with coryza, and cough may point to a viral aetiology.

Presentation: pain on swallowing; fever; headache; tonsillar exudates (Figure 7.2, 📖 p.121); nausea and vomiting; abdominal pain.

Differential diagnosis: glandular fever especially in teenagers with persistent sore throat.

Management: 90% patients recover in <1 wk without treatment. Advise analgesia and antipyretics (e.g. paracetamol and/or ibuprofen), ↑ fluid intake and salt-water gargles. Consider delayed prescription for antibiotics (e.g. penicillin V or erythromycin for 5–10 d) if no improvement in 2–3 d.

Complications of sore throat: all rare:
- *Quinsy (peritonsillar abscess):* usually occurs in adults. *Signs:* unilateral peritonsillar swelling, difficulty swallowing (even saliva) and trismus (difficulty opening jaw). Admit for IV antibiotics ± incision and drainage.
- *Retropharyngeal abscess:* occurs in children. *Signs:* inability to swallow, fever. Admit for IV antibiotics ± incision and drainage.
- *Rheumatic fever.*
- *Glomerulonephritis.*

Scarlet fever: Gp.A haemolytic streptococcus infection with 2–4 d incubation period.

Presentation: fever, malaise, headache, tonsillitis, rash—fine punctate erythema sparing face, 'scarlet' facial flushing, strawberry tongue (initially white turning red by 3rd/4th day).

Management: Penicillin V for 10 d. Complications (rheumatic fever and glomerulonephritis) are rare.

Glandular fever (infectious mononucleosis): consider in teenagers or young adults presenting with sore throat lasting >1 wk. Caused by Epstein–Barr virus (EBV). Spread by droplet infection and direct contact ('kissing disease') and has a 4–14 d incubation period.

Presentation: sore throat, malaise, fatigue, lymphadenopathy, enlarged spleen, palatal petechiae, rash (10–20%). If suspected confirm diagnosis with blood test (FBC and monospot/Paul Bunnell).

Management: advise rest, fluids, and regular paracetamol; try salt water gargles; consider a short course of prednisolone for severe symptoms; treat 2° infection with antibiotics; counsel re the possibility of prolonged symptoms (up to several months).

⚠ DON'T prescribe amoxicillin as it causes a severe rash.

Complications: 2° infections; rash with amoxicillin; hepatitis; jaundice; pneumonitis; neurological disturbances (rare).

Table 7.2 Common childhood viral infections. For all these infections, management is supportive with paracetamol, fluids ± antibiotics for 2° infection. Teething gels, e.g. Calgel® may sooth mouth lesions in hand, foot and mouth disease

Condition	Duration	Main symptoms
Viral upper respiratory tract infection (URTI) e.g. *rhinovirus*	4–7 d	*Incubation:* 3–10 d. *Symptoms:* coryza, runny eyes and malaise ± mild pyrexia ± non-specific maculo papular rash.
Influenza		📖 p.86
Glandular fever		📖 p.119
Croup		📖 p.76
Measles[ND]	10 d	*Incubation:* 10–14 d. *Early symptoms:* fever, conjunctivitis, cough, coryza, LNs. *Later symptoms:* Koplik's spots (tiny white spots on bright red background found on buccal mucosa of cheeks), rash (florid maculo-papular appears after 4 d—becomes confluent). *Complications:* bronchopneumonia, otitis media, stomatitis, corneal ulcers, gastroenteritis, appendicitis, encephalitis (1:1000 affected children), subacute sclerosing panencephalitis (rare).
Rubella[ND] (German measles)	10 d	*Incubation:* 14–21 d. *Symptoms:* mild and may pass unrecognized. Fever, LNs (including suboccipital nodes), pink maculopapular rash which lasts 3 d. *Complications:* birth defects if infected in pregnancy; arthritis (adolescents); thrombocytopenia (rare); encephalitis (rare).
Mumps[ND]	10 d	*Incubation:* 16–21 d. *Symptoms:* subclinical infection is common. Fever, malaise, tender enlargement of 1 or both parotids ± submandibular glands. *Complications:* aseptic meningitis; epididymo-orchitis; pancreatitis.
Roseola infantum	4–7 d	Child <2 y. *Symptoms:* high fever, sore throat and lymphadenopathy, macular rash appears after 3–4 d when fever ↓
Erythema infectiosum* (Fifth disease or slapped cheek) *Parvovirus*	4–7 d	*Symptoms:* erythematous maculopapular rash starting on the face ('slapped cheeks'), reticular, 'lacy' rash on trunk and limbs, mild fever, arthralgia (rare)

Table 7.2 (contd.)

Condition	Duration	Main symptoms
Hand, foot and mouth disease *Coxsackie virus*	5–7 d	*Symptoms:* oral blisters/ulcers, red-edged vesicles on hands and feet, mild fever.
Chickenpox[†] Herpes zoster virus	<14 d	Incubation: 10–21 d. Infectious for 1–2 d before rash appears. Symptoms: rash ± fever. Spots appear in crops for 5–7 d on skin/mucus membranes and progress from macule → papule → vesicle then dry and scab over. Infectious 5d. after rash appears. *Complications:* eczema herpeticum; encephalitis (cerebellar symptoms are most common); pneumonia.

* Pregnant women in contact with parvovirus infection—risk of infection in pregnancy ≈1/400—risk for a non-immune mother with a child who has Fifth disease (slapped cheek) ≈50–90%. Maternal infection results in 4% ↑ miscarriage (<20 wk gestation). Infection between 9 and 20 wk may also cause anaemia of the foetus (3% of those infected). Hydrops fetalis develops 2–17 wk afterwards. If known contact check immune status ± refer for foetal monitoring.

† Non-immune immunosuppressed patients, pregnant women or neonates with significant exposure to chickenpox or shingles, should receive zoster immunoglobulin (VZ-Ig) as soon as possible (<3 d after contact). Check antibody levels if immune status is unknown.

Advice for parents:

- Fever is part of the body's response to infection. Fever in itself, unless very high (over 41.5°C), is not harmful so does not necessarily need treatment.
- Childhood infections may make your child feel uncomfortable and can be helped by giving paracetamol or ibuprofen (follow the instructions on the bottle and don't exceed the recommended dose; aspirin should not be given to children under 16 years old); removing warm clothing and blankets; and sponging with luke warm water
- Children should drink plenty of fluids. If your child is hungry, he or she can eat but often children with infections go off their food.

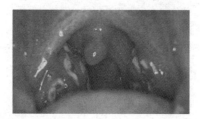

Fig. 7.2 Acute tonsillitis.

Kawasaki disease: epidemiology suggests an infectious aetiology but cause is, as yet, unknown. *Incidence in the UK:* 3.4/100 000 children aged <5 y.

Diagnosis
- There is no diagnostic test and many cases are missed.
- Diagnosis is based on clinical criteria—Table 7.3.
- Difficulty arises due to the similarity of features of Kawasaki disease with those of many other childhood infections and the possibility of atypical presentation of Kawasaki disease.
- Remain alert to the possibility of the diagnosis in any child—particularly if very miserable or with fever for >5 d. Poor response to antipyretics heightens suspicion.

Less characteristic features:
- Rhinorrhoea
- Cough
- Abdominal pain
- Vomiting
- Diarrhoea
- Pain/swelling of joints
- CNS involvement
- Jaundice
- Sterile pyuria

Complications
- Coronary arteritis with formation of aneurysms (20–30% untreated patients).
- In the acute phase these may cause thrombosis within an aneurysm, MI or dysrhythmias and even death.
- Long-term morbidity results from scarring of coronary arteries, intimal thickening, and accelerated atherosclerosis.

Management: If suspected refer for urgent paediatric assessment. Early treatment (<10 d after onset) with IV immunoglobulin and aspirin ↓ incidence and severity of aneurysm formation as well as giving symptom relief. The role of treatment after this time is unclear though IV immunoglobulin is often given >10 d after onset of symptoms if there is evidence of ongoing inflammation.

Table 7.3 Diagnostic criteria for Kawasaki disease

Presence of ≥5 of the following:

- Fever for ≥5 d
- Bilateral (non-purulent) conjunctivitis
- Polymorphous rash
- Changes in lips and mouth:
  - Reddened, dry, or cracked lips
  - Strawberry tongue
  - Diffuse redness of oral or pharyngeal mucosa
- Changes in extremities:
  - Reddening of palms or soles
  - Indurative oedema of hands or feet
  - Desquamation of skin of hands, feet, and groin (in convalescence)
- Cervical lymphadenopathy: >15 mm diameter. Usually unilateral, single, non-purulent, and painful

Exclusion of diseases with similar presentation:

- Staphylococcal infection (such as scalded skin syndrome, toxic shock syndrome)
- Streptococcal infection (e.g. scarlet fever, toxic shock-like syndrome)
- Rickettsial disease
- Leptospirosis
- Stevens–Johnson syndrome
- Drug reaction
- Measles and other viral exanthems
- Juvenile rheumatoid arthritis

❶ Throat carriage of group A streptococcus does not exclude Kawasaki disease.

☼ Sudden infant death syndrome

~1:1500 babies/y are found unexpectedly dead in the 1st year of life in the UK. These deaths are most common in winter months and at night (midnight–9a.m.). An identifiable cause for the death can be found for 1:10 deaths—the rest remain unexplained ('*cot deaths*'). Theories include cardiac arrhythmia and apnoeic attacks. *Peak age: 1–4 mo, ♂>♀.*

Risk factors for cot death

- Baby sleeping face down
- Smoking (mother and other family members)
- Overheating
- Minor intercurrent illness
- Twin or multiple pregnancy
- Low birth weight
- Social disadvantage
- Young mother
- Large numbers of siblings

Management

If you are the first person contacted:

- Check an ambulance is on its way and go immediately to the scene. If in doubt, start resuscitation. Continue until the baby gets to hospital.
- If it is clear the baby is dead and can't be resuscitated, inform the parents sympathetically. Contact the police/coroner. Arrange for the baby to be taken to A&E, not to a mortuary. Contact the paediatrician designated for cot deaths who may wish to see the baby and parents as soon as they get to A&E.
- Take a brief history and record the circumstances of death (e.g. position when found, bedding, vomit, etc.) immediately. Your notes might be helpful later. Spend time listening to the parents. Mention the baby by name and don't be afraid to express your sorrow.
- If the baby is a twin, the surviving twin is at ↑ risk of cot death and should be admitted to hospital for observation.

If you learn later that a baby has died: consider:

- A prompt visit to express sympathy and stress that no one is to blame. There may be some anger directed towards you as often babies have been seen in general practice within a few days or weeks of the death. Do not be defensive or become angry.
- Explain about formalities—necessary post-mortems and coroner's inquests, arranging a funeral, registering the death, etc.
- Discuss suppression of lactation if breast feeding—prescribe cabergoline 250 mcgm bd for 2 d if required.
- Encourage taking photographs of the baby, and other mementoes, i.e. lock of hair, hand and foot prints.

❶ Babies who die at <28 d of age require a special death certificate

Follow-up

- Cancel outstanding appointments for the baby (e.g. developmental screening, immunizations) and inform other involved health/social care professionals.

- Review within a few days. Advise parents about likely grief reactions—guilt, anger, ↓ appetite, sleeplessness, hearing the baby cry. Don't forget siblings—they can be deeply affected too. Continue regular review as long as it is needed and wanted. Be sensitive to anniversaries. Watch for serious psychiatric illness.
- Ensure parents have received written information about cot death, including details of self-help organizations and helplines. Consider referral for counselling—ideal timing for referral varies.
- Ensure you get a copy of the post mortem findings and try to attend the case discussion, which should be held ~1 mo after death.
- Parents should have an opportunity to speak to a consultant paediatrician about the death.
- Refer for specialist obstetric assessment early in the next pregnancy and make sure parents are put in touch with the Care of Next Infant (CONI) scheme. Discuss the use of apnoea alarms.

Apnoea alarms: commonly issued to or purchased by parents if they are worried about the risk of cot death. An apnoea alarm cannot be useful unless parents are taught basic life support to a proficient standard. An alarm should not be supplied without this training. There is no evidence that apnoea alarms prevent cot deaths.

Near-miss cot deaths: parents may rush a child to A&E or the GP after an episode of pallor ± floppiness. Parents may have attempted mouth to mouth resuscitation before the baby starts to respond to them or may have simply touched the baby or lifted him up and received a response. Usually there are no residual symptoms or signs.

Management: difficult. Parents may have misinterpreted normal irregularities in sleep or the child might be unwell and have a physical cause for symptoms, e.g. early stages of a viral infection. Usually parents are very anxious by the time you see the child. Take a careful history and examine the child from top to toe. Treat any cause of symptoms found. Be as reassuring as possible and play down anxieties.

⚠ If the child has any risk factors for cot death, comes from a difficult social background or parents are unable to cope following the episode—admit the child for observation and further assessment.

Further information and parent support

Foundation for the Study of Infant Deaths (FSID) Guidelines for general practitioners when a baby dies suddenly and unexpectedly (2003); information; support; administration of the CONI scheme 🖳 www.sids.org.uk

Child bereavement trust ☎ 0845 357 1000 🖳 www.childbereavement.org.uk

Child death helpline. ☎ 0800 282 986 🖳 www.childdeathhelpline.org.uk

⊛ Child abuse and neglect

Defined as depriving children of their Human Rights. These are:
- *Being healthy:* enjoying good physical and mental health and living a healthy lifestyle
- *Staying safe:* being protected from harm and neglect
- *Enjoying and achieving:* developing broad skills for adulthood
- *Making a positive contribution:* to the community and society
- *Economic well-being:* overcoming disadvantages to achieve their full potential

Statistics: ~3/100 children are abused each year in the UK; there were 4109 reported offences of cruelty or neglect of children in England and Wales in 2002/3 and every year, ~30 000 children's names are added to the child protection register in England alone.

Presentation: *always* have a high index of suspicion. Suspect abuse if:
- The child discloses it
- The story is inconsistent with injuries found
- There is late presentation after an injury or lack of concern about the injury by the parent(s)
- Presentation to an unknown doctor
- Accompanying adult is not the parent or guardian
- Sibling has been a victim of abuse
- Reluctance to allow the child to be examined
- Characteristic injuries—look for marks consistent with cigarette burns; scalds (especially if symmetrical or doughnut shaped on buttocks); finger mark or bite mark bruises; perineal bruising or anogenital injury; linear marks consistent with whipping; buckle or belt marks
- Multiple injuries or old injuries coexistent with new
- Unlikely sites for injuries, e.g. mouth, ears, genitalia, eyes
- Behaviour of the child is suggestive: e.g. withdrawn, 'frozen watchfulness', sexually precocious behaviour, abnormal interaction between child and parents, unwilling to speak about the injury etc.
- Vaginal discharge, sexually transmitted disease or recurrent UTI in any child <14 y
- Failure to thrive, developmental delay and/or behavioural problems: neglect and/or emotional abuse are included in the differential diagnosis of failure to thrive and developmental delay. Any type of abuse may result in behavioural problems.

Risk factors for child abuse

Parent/carer factors:
- Mental illness
- Substance/alcohol abuse
- Being abused themselves as children or adults
- Ongoing physical illness
- Learning disabilities
- Unemployment/ impoverished living conditions

Child factors:
- History of sibling abuse
- Learning, behaviour or physical problems
- Unplanned pregnancy/premature birth
- Poor attachment to parents/carers
- Environment high in criticism
- 'Looked after' children

Table 7.4 Classification of child abuse

PHYSICAL	EMOTIONAL
Hitting, shaking, throwing, burning, suffocating, poisoning, including factitious or induced illness	The child is made to feel worthless, afraid, unloved or inadequate (e.g. if developmentally inappropriate expectations are imposed)

NEGLECT	SEXUAL
Failure to meet the child's basic needs, allowing the child to be exposed to danger	Forcing/enticing a child to take part in sexual activities—may involve physical contact, or production of pornographic material

❶ In practice there is often overlap and >1 type of abuse may co-occur.

⚠ **Special circumstances to watch out for**

- Circumcision of female infants
- Forced marriage of minors (<16 y)

Both these practices are illegal in the UK, but it is not uncommon for children to be taken abroad to be circumcised/married. If you suspect this might be going to happen to any patient of yours, inform social services and/or the police immediately.

How to safeguard children with confidence

- Make sure you are familiar with the practice and local child protection procedures.
- Make sure you attend child protection training regularly
- Share your concerns with colleagues and try to use shared documentation and computer templates as much as possible.

Immediate action
- Wherever possible, arrange for another health professional to be present during the consultation.
- Take a history from any accompanying adult. If possible also take a history from the child alone too.
- Examine the child. Ask for an explanation for any injuries noted.
- Keep thorough notes—recording dates and times, history given, injuries noted and any explanation of those injuries.

⚠ Welfare of the child is *paramount*—not to report abuse is to collude with the abuser. Do *not* perform a forensic-type examination unless you are trained to do so and be careful not to ask leading questions which might contaminate the evidence.

Further action: depends on nature of the suspected abuse, suspected abuser (e.g. if someone outside the home is suspected, the child is safe to return home), nature of the injuries and response of the parents. Be familiar with and follow local guidelines and practice policy. *Options are:*
- Hospital admission—protects the child and allows full assessment.
- Liaison with social services child protection team (on-call 24 h/d).
- If admission is refused, contact social services to arrange a Place of Safety Order, or the police to take the child into police protection.
- Contact social services if your observations and discussions lead you to feel that this is a child protection issue and follow the referral up in 48 h with a written referral—you should receive confirmation of your referral in 1–3 working days.
- You can also refer directly to the police particularly if you feel emergency action may be required to protect the child.

Difficult issues in safeguarding children
- Confidentiality of medical information
- Sharing information with parents and carers
- Fear of damaging future relationships with the family
- Fear of causing family disruption
- Fear of dealing with other agencies, e.g. police and social services
- Fear of being mistaken in ones' suspicions
- Fear of missing abuse
- Fear of attending court
- Fear of negative peer review.

Refugee children: have special problems and needs. *Consider:*
- *Language barriers*—consider the use of professional interpreters even if the child is with an English speaking carer.
- *Cultural and religious issues*—if in doubt, ask
- *Physical needs*—health needs are diverse depending on country of origin and previous level of health care. Consider infectious diseases, e.g. hepatitis B, HIV, TB and malaria. Check immunization status.
- *Psychological needs*—many child refugees have traumatic backgrounds. Approach children with sensitivity and consider involving specialist child psychiatric services and specialist refugee support services early.
- *Family*—some children will have left family members behind. The Red Cross or Red Crescent can help with tracing (🖳 www.redcross.org.uk).

Step 1	Step 2	Step 3	Step 4
Recognition	**Reporting**	**Enquiry and assessment of risk**	**Intervention**
Health professionals either identify or suspect a situation where a child may be at risk of abuse or neglect.	Suspicions are reported or discussed with social services, police and/or child protection agencies.	Concerns and allegations are explored, information is gathered and risk to children determined.	Consists of supportive and rehabilitation measures in order to enable child development.
	Concerns regarding a family become 'public'— this is often the threshold at which those in primary care hesitate and step hesitate and step brink.	A multi-agency approach is usually employed.	

Fig. 7.3 The 4-step approach to safeguarding children.

⚠ This guidance appears simple—and *is* when abuse is overt—but often it is *difficult* to decide if a child is being abused. If you have worries but cannot justify them sufficiently to invoke child protection procedures:

• Check via social services whether the child is on the 'at risk' register
• Check notes of siblings and other family members to see if there has been any suggestion of abuse in the family before
• Discuss your worries with the health visitor and/or other involved members of the primary health care team.

If any of these sources ↑ your suspicion, you may be justified in investigating further or invoking child protection measures at that point.

If you are still unsure what to do, record your worries and the reasons for them in the child's notes and alert all other involved members of the practice team. Review whenever that child is seen again in the practice

Further information

DoH 🖳 www.dh.gov.uk
• Working together to safeguard children (1998)
• What to do if you're worried a child is being abused (2003)
RCGP *Carter & Bannon.* The Role of Primary Care in the protection of children from abuse and neglect (2003) 🖳 www.rcgp.org.uk
Department for Education and skills Every Child matters (2004) 🖳 www.everychildmatters.gov.uk
The refugee council 🖳 www.refugeecouncil.org.uk

Neurological emergencies

:O: The fitting patient

When the call for assistance is received: instruct the attendant to:
• stay with the fitting patient
• move anything from the vicinity of the patient that might cause injury
• turn the patient on to his/her side.

If the patient is a child, suspect a febrile cause and advise the attendant to cool the child by stripping off layers of clothing and tepid sponging.

⚠ Management of a major fit

• Ensure that the airway is clear
• Turn the patient into the recovery position (Figure 8.1)
• Prevent onlookers from restraining the fitting patient
• Do not give drugs for the 1st 10 min—the fit is likely to stop spontaneously
• After 10 min treat with diazepam 5–10 mg IV or pr (5 mg if 2–3 y or elderly; 2.5 mg if <2y)
• If the fit is not controlled treat as status epilepticus.

Admit any patient with a fit if:

• there is suspicion that the fit is secondary to other illness, e.g. meningitis, subdural haematoma
• the patient doesn't recover completely after the fit (other than feeling sleepy)
• status epilepticus

Status epilepticus: if >1 seizure without the patient regaining consciousness or fitting continues >20 min:
• Give diazepam 5–10 mg IV or pr (5 mg if 2–3 y or elderly; 2.5 mg if <2 y).
• Repeat every 15 min until fits are controlled.
• Check BM to exclude low blood sugar.
• Arrange immediate admission even if fits are controlled.

Follow-up

• Refer any adult who has a first fit to neurology for urgent assessment.
• Refer any child who has a first fit not related to fever to paediatrics for urgent assessment.

Febrile convulsions: 📖 p.138–141.

Delirium tremens (DTs): major alcohol withdrawal symptoms usually occur 2–3 d after an alcoholic has stopped drinking.

Features

• *General:* fever, tachycardia, ↑BP, ↑ respiratory rate
• *Psychiatric:* vivid visual and tactile hallucinations, acute confusional state, apprehension
• *Neurological:* tremor, fits, fluctuating level of consciousness.

⚠ **Action:** DTs have 15% mortality and always warrant emergency hospital admission.

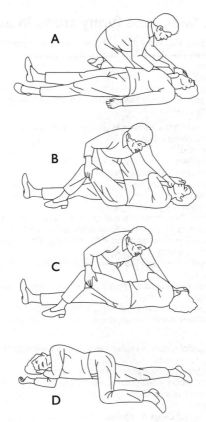

Fig. 8.1 The recovery position.

Further information

NICE ☐ www.nice.org.uk
- The epilepsies: diagnosis and management of the epilepsies in adults and children in primary and secondary care (2004)
- Referral guidelines for suspected cancer—quick reference guide (2005)

◉ Fits, faints and funny turns in adults

Blackouts, faints and funny turns are all common presentations. The major questions that should be asked seeing an individual who has had a funny turn are:
- Is it epilepsy?
- If it is epilepsy, then what kind?
- If it is not epilepsy, then is there another serious underlying cause, e.g. heart disease?

History: a good history from the patient and ideally from a witness is essential in the correct diagnosis. Ask:
- What happened?
- When and where? Particularly, did it start during sleep?
- Were there any precipitating events?
- Were there any warning signs? e.g. aura, feeling going to faint, etc.
- Does the patient remember the whole episode? If not, which bits are missing and how long are the gaps?
- Did the patient lose consciousness? Quite frequently patients describe episodes of dizziness or unsteadiness/falling as 'funny turns'.
- Did the patient jerk his/her limbs? If so, was the jerking generalized or restricted to one area of the body?
- What did the patient look like during the attack? An eye witness account is helpful.
- Did anything else happen during the attack? e.g. tongue biting, incontinence.
- What happened after the attack? Was the patient conscious straight away? Was there disorientation, drowsiness or headache?

Also check
- General medical history, including cardiac history and history of other neurological symptoms
- Psychiatric history? Anxiety, depression, panic attacks
- Past medical history—birth trauma, febrile convulsions in childhood, significant head injury and/or meningitis/encephalitis
- Family history—epilepsy
- Substance abuse? Drugs or alcohol.

Examination: complete general and neurological examination. Particularly check for:
- *Skin changes*—café-au-lait spots (neurofibromatosis); adenoma sebaceum (tuberous sclerosis); trigeminal capillary haemangioma (Sturge–Weber syndrome)
- *Cardiovascular abnormalities*—heart rate and rhythm, murmurs, carotid bruits, BP
- *Focal neurological deficits*—suggest presence of a structural neurological lesion.

Differential diagnosis: Figure 8.2.

Funny turns in small children: 📖 p.136.

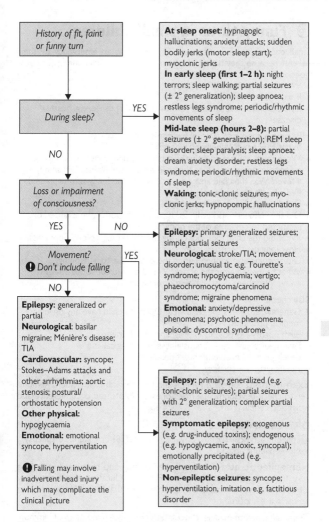

Fig. 8.2 Differential diagnosis of fits, faints and funny turns.

👁 **Funny turns in small children**

Small children are often brought to the GP as an emergency by their parents because they have had a funny turn. As in adults, the major questions are:

- Was the episode a fit?
- If so, what caused it?
- If not, then is there another serious underlying cause, e.g. heart disease?

History: a good history from a witness is essential. Ask:

- What happened? When and where?
- Were there any precipitating events or warning signs something was going to happen? e.g. Does the child have a viral illness? Did s/he have a fever? Was the child angry or upset when the funny turn happened? Did s/he hit his/her head?
- Did the child lose consciousness?
- Did the child jerk his/her limbs? If so, was the jerking generalized or restricted to one area of the body?
- What did the child look like during the attack? e.g. colour, floppiness.
- How long did the attack last?
- Did anything else happen during the attack? e.g. tongue biting.
- What happened after the attack? Was the child conscious straight away? Was there disorientation or drowsiness?

Also check:

- General history—is the child well? Does the child have any ongoing medical problems?
- Birth history—problems in pregnancy, birth trauma.
- Past medical history—serious illness, neurological and/or developmental problems, heart problems.
- Family history—epilepsy.

Examination: complete general and neurological examination. Remember to check developmental milestones and plot head circumference and weight on centile chart.

Differential diagnosis

- Epileptic attacks—febrile convulsion (📖 p.138) or childhood epilepsy.
- Non-epileptic attacks.

Non-epileptic attacks: usually self-limiting and harmless but can be very frightening for parents/carers. Parental education about the likely duration and cause of attacks and reassurance that the child will come to no harm are important.

Simple blue breath-holding attacks: onset usually >6 mo of age. Common. Provoked by frustration or upset. *Signs:* +ve valsalva manoeuvre, cyanosis, stiffening and coma. No treatment needed—spontaneous recovery. Most children 'grow out' of the attacks by 3y.

White reflex asystolic (anoxic) attacks: may start before 6 mo but most common from 6 mo to 2 y. Usually triggered by minor injury or anxiety. *Signs:* vagal asystole, pallor, rapid coma, stiffening, upward eye movement ± urinary incontinence. No treatment needed—spontaneous recovery.

Reflex syncope or vasovagal attacks ('faints'): common. Peripheral vaso-dilation, bradycardia and venous pooling → postural hypotension. Often cause is unclear though ♀>♂. *Known precipitants:* fright (e.g. during vene-section) or emotion. *Features:*
- *Prodrome*—dizziness, visual disturbance, nausea, sweating, ringing in the ears, a sinking feeling and yawning
- *Faint*—extreme pallor, momentary unconsciousness (with fall to the floor if standing ± tonic-clonic jerks if held upright)
- *Rapid recovery.*

No treatment is needed—reassure.

Others causes are rare in children but include:
- Cardiac arrhythmias—the NSF for coronary heart disease recommends all children with recurrent loss of consciousness or collapse on exertion are referred for paediatric cardiology assessment.
- Hyperventilation
- Benign monoclonus of infancy
- Benign paroxysmal vertigo
- Sleep phenomena
- Hypoglycaemia
- Munchausen syndrome by proxy

Further information
NICE The epilepsies: the diagnosis and management of the epilepsies in adults and children in primary and secondary care (2004) ▣ www.nice.org.uk
NSF for coronary hart disease (2005) ▣ www.dh.gov.uk

⊛ Febrile convulsions

A febrile convulsion is a seizure occurring in a child aged 6 mo–5 y (peak age 18 mo), associated with fever arising from infection or inflammation outside the central nervous system, in a child who is otherwise neurologically normal[1]. 2–4% of all children have a febrile convulsion.

Classification

- *Simple febrile convulsions:* isolated, generalized, tonic-clonic seizures lasting <10–15 min.
- *Complex febrile convulsions:* last 15–30 min, or are focal, or recur during the febrile illness, or are not followed by full consciousness within 1 h.

Causes: in ↓ order of frequency:
- viral infections
- otitis media
- tonsillitis
- UTI
- gastroenteritis
- lower respiratory tract infection
- meningitis
- post-immunization.

Assessment: by the time the GP arrives, the febrile convulsion is usually over, so diagnosis is based on a history of short, generalized tonic-clonic seizure in a febrile child.

Examination and investigation: the main concern when assessing children who have had a febrile convulsion is to detect and manage bacterial meningitis (☐ p.148). Check temperature, assess level of consciousness and examine for a source of infection (see causes above). If there is no obvious cause and the child is not being admitted, check an MSU for urinary tract infection.

⚠ Complex are more likely than simple febrile convulsions to be provoked by a serious condition. Suspect serious pathology if a child has:
- had a prolonged febrile convulsion
- had a focal febrile convulsion, or
- not recovered within an hour of a febrile convulsion.

Differential diagnosis

- *Epilepsy*
- *Any other cause of convulsion:*
  - meningitis or encephalitis
  - cerebral palsy with intercurrent infection
  - hypoglycaemia
  - neurodegenerative disorders
  - poisoning (e.g. inadvertent drug ingestion)
  - NAI

---

1 Offringa and Moyer (2001) *BMJ* 323(7321) pp.1111–1114.

Management of the fitting patient: 📖 p.132.

Management of febrile convulsions: 📖 p.140.

Frequently asked questions about febrile convulsions

What is the risk of recurrence after a febrile convulsion?

Febrile convulsions recur in subsequent febrile illnesses in ~30% of children—9% have >3 seizures. Recurrence is most common in the year following the first febrile convulsion. Recurrence is more likely if:

- First febrile convulsion aged <15 mo.
- First febrile convulsion is complex.
- Family history of febrile convulsions or epilepsy in a 1st-degree relative.
- Child attends day nursery (↑ frequency of febrile illnesses).

Is there an increased risk of epilepsy after febrile convulsion?

Rarely—1% of children having a febrile convulsion go on to develop epilepsy (compared to 0.4% children who have not had a febrile convulsion). Risk ↑ if any of the following features are present:

- Neurological abnormalities or developmental delay before the onset of febrile convulsions
- Atypical seizures
- Family history of epilepsy
- Complex convulsions.

Are there long-term complications after febrile convulsions?

Long-term adverse effects are rare. There is no evidence of subsequent impaired intelligence or poorer academic achievement but there is a slightly increased risk of epilepsy.

Is immunization contraindicated after febrile convulsion?

There is evidence to suggest immunizations do not ↑ risk of recurrent febrile convulsions.[1] Immunization is not contraindicated.

Management: most children do *not* need admission.

Admit if:
- The child was drowsy before the seizure
- The child is irritable, systemically unwell or 'toxic' and/or the cause of the fever is unclear
- Petechial rash
- Symptoms/signs of meningitis—🕮 p.148
- Recent/current treatment with antibiotics (may mask symptoms/signs of meningitis)
- Age <18 mo (meningitis may present with non-specific signs)
- The cause of the fever requires hospital management in its own right
- Complex convulsion
- Early review by a doctor is not possible
- Inadequate home circumstances
- Carer anxious or unable to cope

For children not being admitted
- Reassure parents/carers that febrile convulsions do not harm the child.
- Advise on controlling fever in the future: an antipyretic, e.g. paracetamol or ibuprofen syrup, cool clothing. If not managing to lower temperature with these measures, fan the child or sponge with lukewarm water.
- Teach parents to manage a recurrent convulsion: recovery position, nothing forced into mouth.
- Recommend that immunization schedules be completed.
- Advise the parents/carers to seek urgent medical help if the child deteriorates in any way, fits again or they are worried.
- Arrange early review, e.g. later the same day or the following morning.

Consider referral to paediatrics or paediatric neurology if:
- Diagnosis of febrile convulsion is in doubt.
- Febrile convulsions have been frequent, severe and/or complex and prophylactic treatment might be indicated.
- The child is at ↑ risk of epilepsy, e.g. coexistent neurological or developmental conditions; history of epilepsy in 1st degree relative.
- The parents/carers are still anxious despite reassurance or request a specialist opinion.

Prophylactic measures: Prescribe under consultant direction only.
- *Rectal diazepam:* may prevent febrile convulsions in subsequent illness if given at the onset of a febrile episode. Rectal diazepam is safe for home use provided parents are properly educated about its use.
- *Continuous prophylaxis:* use of anticonvulsants on a regular basis to prevent frequent febrile convulsions is controversial. In general benefits are outweighed by risks.

Information for parents about febrile convulsions
What are febrile convulsions?
A febrile convulsion or fit happens when normal brain activity is disturbed when a child has a fever. It usually occurs without warning. During the fit your child may:

- become stiff or floppy
- become unconscious or unaware of their surroundings
- display jerking or twitching movements
- have difficulty breathing.

Febrile convulsions are frightening to watch, but they are not harmful to your child, don't cause brain damage, and will not cause your child to die.

What happens after a febrile convulsion?
Your child will become tired for up to an hour after the fit. If your child remains sleepy or is difficult to rouse after sleep, seek medical attention.

Will my child have another febrile convulsion?
Possibly—febrile convulsions may recur. About 1 in 3 children who have had a febrile convulsion will have another. The risk of another febrile convulsion decreases with time as the child gets older. Immunization is still advised after a febrile convulsion, even if, as rarely happens, the febrile convulsion followed an immunization.

Are febrile convulsions the same as epilepsy?
No—febrile convulsions are not epilepsy. Rarely, in about 1 in 100 children who have had more than one febrile convulsion, epilepsy can develop later.

How can I prevent fevers which cause convulsions?
Controlling fever eases symptoms. It does not prevent febrile convulsions. A high temperature can be reduced by:

- Giving paracetamol or ibuprofen—read the instructions on the packet carefully and only give your child the recommended dose for his age
- Removing excessive clothing or bedding—in the home this usually means stripping your child down to underwear or nappy.

What should I do if my child has another convulsion?
Remember, most fits stop within a couple of minutes without treatment.

- Stay calm
- Look at your watch or a clock and time the convulsion
- Don't try to restrain your child or put anything in his mouth
- Stay with your child and lie him on his side
- Loosen tight clothing from around his neck and move objects away that may cause injury
- Ring your GP or NHS direct after the convulsion has stopped.

Call an ambulance if:

- The fit lasts for more than 5 min
- Another fit starts up after the first one stops
- Your child has difficulty breathing or looks particularly unwell.

Headache and migraine

Common presenting complaint. The skill lies in deciding which headaches are benign needing no intervention, and which require action.

History

- *Does the patient have >1 type of headache?* Take a separate history for each.
- *Time:* When did the headaches start? New or recently changed headache calls for especially careful assessment. How often do they happen? Do they have any pattern? (e.g. constant, episodic, daily) How long do they last? Why is the patient consulting now?
- *Character:* nature and quality, site and spread of the pain. Associated symptoms, e.g. nausea/vomiting, visual disturbance, photophobia, neurological symptoms.
- *Cause:* predisposing and/or trigger factors; aggravating and/or relieving factors; family history.
- *Response:* details of medication used (type, dose, frequency, timing). What does the patient do? e.g. can the patient continue work?
- *Health between attacks:* Do the headaches go completely or does the patient still feel unwell between attacks?
- *Anxieties and concerns* of the patient.

Examination

- In acute, severe headache, examine for purpuric skin rash
- BP
- Brief neurological examination including fundi, visual acuity and gait
- Palpation of the temporal region/sinuses for tenderness
- Examination of the neck
- *In young children* measure head circumference and plot on a centile chart.

Investigation: often not needed. Consider ESR if temporal arteritis is suspected.

Management: direct treatment at cause.

Differential diagnosis: Table 8.1.

❶ ↑BP may cause acute or chronic headache.

☼ **Meningism:** headache, stiff neck and photophobia. Associated with meningitis ▣ p.148. May also be seen with encephalitis and SAH.

◉ **Facial pain:** treat the cause. *Common causes include:* trigeminal neuralgia; temporomandibular joint disorders; dental disorders; sinusitis; migrainous neuralgia; shingles and post-herpetic neuralgia.

No cause is found in many patients—it is then termed *atypical facial pain.* Atypical facial pain may respond to simple analgesia with paracetamol or a NSAID. If this fails, try nerve painkillers, e.g. amitriptyline nocte. Refer those with troublesome symptoms to ENT, maxillofacial surgery or neurology.

Table 8.1 Differential diagnosis of headache

	Cause	Features	Management
Acute new headache	Meningitis	Fever, photophobia, stiff neck, rash, photophobia	IV or IM penicillin V and immediate admission (📖 p.148)
	Encephalitis	Fever, confusion, ↓ conscious level	Immediate admission (📖 p.148)
	Subarachnoid haemorrhage	'Thunder-clap' or very sudden onset headache ± stiff neck.	Immediate admission (📖 p.144)
	Head injury	Bruising/injury; ↓ conscious level, periods lucidity, amnesia	Consider admission (📖 p.222)
	Acute febrile illness	Fever and symptoms of underlying cause, e.g. URTI, tonsillitis	Treat underlying cause
	Acute sinusitis	Tender over sinuses ± history of URTI.	📖 p.144
	Dental caries	Facial pain ± tenderness	Consider antibiotics. Refer to dentist
	Tropical illness	History of travel, fever	Consider admission
Acute recurrent headache	Migraine	Aura, visual disturbance, nausea/vomiting, triggers.	📖 p.144
	Cluster headache	Nightly pain in 1 eye for 2–3 mo then pain free for >1 y	📖 p.146
	Exertional or coital headache	Suggested by history of association.	NSAID, or propranolol before attacks
	Trigeminal neuralgia	Intense stabbing pain lasting seconds in trigeminal nerve distribution.	📖 p.146
	Glaucoma	Red eye, haloes, ↓ visual acuity, pupil abnormality	📖 p.172
Subacute headache	Temporal (giant cell) arteritis	>50 y, scalp tenderness, ↑ ESR, rarely ↓ visual acuity	📖 p.146
Chronic headache	Tension type headache	Band around the head, stress, low mood.	📖 p.147
	Cervicogenic headache	Unilateral or bilateral; band from neck to forehead; scalp tenderness.	📖 p.204
	Medication overuse headache	Rebound headache on stopping analgesics.	📖 p.147
	↑ intracranial pressure	Worse on waking/sneezing, neurological signs (possibly including papilloedema), ↑BP, ↓ pulse rate.	Same day neurology referral or admit
	Paget's disease	>40 y, bowed tibia, ↑ alk phos.	Refer to rheumatology

⚙ **Subarachnoid haemorrhage (SAH):** spontaneous bleeding into the subarachnoid space. Incidence 15/100 000. ♀>♂. Peak age 35–65 y. Frequently fatal. *Causes:*

- No cause (15%)
- Rupture of congenital berry aneurysm (70%)
- Arteriovenous malformation (15%)
- Bleeding disorder
- Mycotic aneurysm 2° to endocarditis (rare)

Risk factors: smoking, alcohol, ↑BP, lack of oestrogen (less common pre-menopause). Berry aneurysms may run in families and are associated with polycystic kidneys, coarctation of the aorta and Ehlers–Danlos syndrome.

Presentation
- Typically presents as a sudden devastating headache—'thunderclap headache'—often occipital.
- Rarely (6%) preceded by a 'sentinel headache' representing a small leak ahead of a larger bleed.
- Vomiting and collapse with loss of consciousness ± fitting ± focal neurology follow.

Examination: may be nothing to find initially. Neck stiffness takes 6 h to develop. In later stages:
- Papilloedema
- Retinal and other intraocular haemorrhages
- Focal neurology
- ↓ level of consciousness

Action: if suspected admit immediately as a medical emergency. Only 1:4 admitted with suspected SAH turn out to have one. In most no cause for the headache is found.

⊛ **Acute sinusitis:** infection of one or more paranasal sinuses (maxillary, frontal, ethmoid or sphenoid). Usually follows a viral URTI though 10% are due to tooth infection.

Presentation: frontal headache/facial pain (may be difficult to distinguish from toothache)—typically worse on movement/bending ± purulent nasal discharge ± fever. Often preceded by URTI.

Management: most sinusitis resolves spontaneously in 7–10 d. Treatment options:
- Advise analgesia (paracetamol ± ibuprofen) and fluids for all patients
- Steam inhalation may help
- Short courses of decongestants may help but there is very little evidence of effectiveness
- Steroid nasal sprays (e.g. beclometasone nasal spray 2 puffs to each nostril bd) may help—evidence of effectiveness is limited.
- Reserve antibiotics for patients with frontal sinusitis, severe symptoms or symptoms persisting >7 d—there is limited evidence of benefit. If prescribing use amoxicillin 250–500 mg tds or erythromycin 250–500 mg qds for 7 d. Doxycycline (200 mg on day 1 then 100 mg od for 6 d) is an alternative.

⊛ **Migraine:** affects 10% of the UK population. ♂:♀ ≈1:2. Caused by disturbance of cerebral blood flow under the influence of 5-HT. Attacks can force the patient to abandon everyday activities for several days.

Clinical picture: 3 common types:
- *Aura*—aura alone with no headache—visual chaos (e.g. zig-zag lines, jumbling of print, dots); hemianopia; hemiparesis; dysphasia; dyspraxia; dysarthria; ataxia (basilar migraine).
- *Classical migraine*—aura lasting 10–30 min followed by unilateral throbbing headache ± nausea/vomiting ± photophobia.
- *Episodic migraine (common migraine)*—unilateral throbbing headache ± nausea/vomiting ± photophobia. No aura—often premenstrual.

Trigger factors: ½ have a trigger for their migraine. Consider:
- *Psychological factors:* stress/relief of stress; anxiety/depression; extreme emotions, e.g. anger or grief.
- *Food factors:* lack of food/infrequent meals; foods containing monosodium glutamate, caffeine and tyramine; specific foods, e.g. chocolate, citrus fruits, cheese; alcohol, especially red wine.
- *Sleep:* overtiredness (physical/mental); changes in sleep patterns (e.g. late nights, weekend lie-in, shift work, holidays); long distance travel.
- *Environmental factors:* loud noise, bright/flickering lights, strong perfume, stuffy atmosphere, VDUs, strong winds, extreme heat/cold.
- *Health factors:* hormonal changes (e.g. monthly periods, COC pill, HRT, the menopause);↑BP; toothache or pain in the eyes, sinuses or neck; unaccustomed physical activity.

Management of an acute attack
- *Advise to rest* in a quiet, dark place and sleep if possible.
- *Analgesia*—dispersible aspirin 900 mg, ibuprofen 400 mg or soluble paracetamol 1 g at 1st signs of an attack ± antiemetic, e.g. domperidone. 20 mg If vomiting consider pr administration, e.g. diclofenac 100 mg pr.
- *Severe attacks*—in addition consider 5HT$_1$ agonists, e.g. sumatriptan 50–100 mg po, 20 mg nasal spray or 6 mg s/cut (not effective if taken before the headache develops—stop 70–85% attacks—start with lowest dose and ↑ as needed—do not give if ergotamine taken <24 h previously).

If called to see a patient with an acute attack:
- Administer IM diclofenac 75 mg ± IM chlorpromazine 25–50 mg.
- Alternatively consider 5HT$_1$ agonist, e.g. sumatriptan unless 2 injections/tablets/nasal sprays already given in last 24 h (or ergotamine in <24 h).
- Admit if becoming dehydrated.

Treatment of recurrence within the same attack: repeat symptomatic treatments within their dose limitations—pre-emptively if recurrence is usual/expected. If using triptans, a 2nd dose may be effective, but repeated dosing can cause rebound headache. Naratriptan and eletriptan are associated with relatively low recurrence rates.

Further information
British Association for the Study of Headache Guidelines for all doctors in the diagnosis and management of migraine and tension type headache (2nd edition—2003) ▣ www.bash.org.uk

Cluster headaches (migrainous neuralgia): clusters of extremely painful headaches focused around 1 eye with associated autonomic symptoms (drooping eyelid, red watery eye, runny or blocked nose). May occur at any age but rare <20 y. ♂:♀ ≈6:1. More common in smokers. Pain lasts up to 1 h and occurs 1–2×/d every day for 4–12 wk then disappears for 1–2 y. Recurrences affect the same side. Onset is often predictable (1–2 h after falling asleep; after alcohol).

Management of an acute attack: give:
- 100% oxygen at a rate of 7–12 l/min if available.
- 5HT₁ agonists, e.g. sumatriptan (6 mg s/cut)—stop ¾ attacks in <15 min.

Follow-up: refer for specialist advice.

ⓔ **Trigeminal neuralgia**
- Paroxysms of intense stabbing, burning or 'electric shock' type pain lasting seconds to minutes in the trigeminal (V) nerve distribution.
- 96% unilateral.
- Mandibular/maxillary >ophthalmic division.
- Between attacks there are no symptoms.
- Frequency of attacks is highly variable ranging from hundreds of attacks/d to remissions lasting years.
- Pain is often provoked by movement of the face (talking, eating, laughing) or by touching the skin (shaving, washing).
- Can occur at any age but more common >50 y; ♀>♂.
- Unknown cause. More common in patients with MS and ♀ with ↑BP.

Management: spontaneous remission may occur.
- Carbamazepine ↓ frequency/intensity of attacks. NNT=1.8. Start at low dose, e.g. 100 mg od/bd and ↑ dose over several weeks until symptoms are controlled. Usual dose ≈200 mg tds. Oxcarbazine is an alternative.
- Gabapentin ↓ frequency and intensity of attacks. Start with 300 mg od on day 1. On day 2 ↑ to 300 mg bd and ↑ again to 300 mg tds on day 3. Increase further according to response to a maximum of 1.8 g daily (in divided doses)

Refer to neurology if:
- <50 y old
- Neurological deficit between attacks
- If treatment with carbamazepine/gabapentin fails—specialist options include lamotrigine, baclofen, phenytoin, or surgical intervention.

⚠ **Temporal arteritis:** unilateral throbbing headache/facial pain and/or scalp tenderness, e.g. on brushing hair, and/or jaw claudication. Visual symptoms include amaurosis fugax, diplopia, and/or sudden loss of vision/blindness.
- *Blood:* ↑ESR (usually >30) ± normocytic anaemia.
- *Temporal artery biopsy:* refer urgently. Biopsy may be -ve even in true cases due to skip lesions. *Do not* withhold treatment while awaiting biopsy—but if taking steroids for ≥2 wk +ve biopsy is less likely.

Management: prescribe prednisolone 1 mg/kg/d (maximum 60 mg od); refer urgently to ophthalmology.

Follow-up
- In all cases, ↓ dose of prednisolone as symptoms allow, e.g. by 2.5 mg every 4 wk until taking 10 mg prednisolone od, then by 1 mg/mo to 5 mg od, then more slowly. Check ESR with dose changes. Stop steroid reduction and recheck ESR if ↑ symptoms. At the start of treatment give osteoporosis prophylaxis and supply with a steroid card.
- Most patients require >2 y of treatment. Relapse is common after stopping treatment (50% if stopped after 2 y). Review diagnosis.

⊚ **Tension type headache:** associated with stress and anxiety and/or functional or structural abnormalities of the head or neck. Prevalence ≈2%. ♀:♂ ≈2:1. Symptoms begin aged <10 y in 15% patients. Prevalence ↓ with age. Family history of similar headaches is common (40%) but twin studies do not suggest a genetic basis. Distinguish between episodic and chronic tension type headache:
- *Episodic:* headache lasting 30 min–7 d and occurring <180 d/y (<15 d/mo).
- *Chronic:* headaches on ≥15 d/mo (≥180 d/y) for ≥6 mo.

In both cases pain:
- Is bilateral, pressing, and/or tightening in quality
- Of mild or moderate intensity
- Does not prohibit activities
- Is not aggravated by routine physical activity
- Is not associated with vomiting
- Is associated with ≥1 of: nausea, photophobia, or phonophobia.

Management
- Reassure no serious underlying pathology.
- Try measures to alleviate stress—relaxation; massage; yoga; exercise. Cognitive therapy is probably effective but not widely available[CE].
- Treat musculoskeletal symptoms with physiotherapy.

Drug therapy: analgesics are of limited value and might make matters worse (see medication overuse headache).
- *Headache <2x/wk:* simple analgesia, e.g. paracetamol, ibuprofen. Avoid codeine-containing preparations.
- *Chronic headache:* amitriptyline 25–75 mg nocte may help. Stop once improvement is maintained for >4–6 mo.

Further information
British Association for the Study of Headache Guidelines for all doctors in the diagnosis and management of migraine and tension type headache (2nd edition—2003) ▣ www.bash.org.uk

⊚ **Medication overuse (analgesic) headache:** persistent headache may develop in patients with other causes of headache, e.g. tension headache or migraine, if they overuse the medication used to treat those conditions. Implicated drugs include: ergotamine, triptans, aspirin, paracetamol and NSAIDs. ♀:♂ ≈3:1. Ask any patient complaining of chronic daily headache (headache >15 d/mo) to give a detailed account of medication use (including OTC)—a diary can be helpful.

Management: aim to ↓ analgesic consumption until <15 d/mo.

☼ Meningitis and encephalitis

Meningitis and encephalitis present in similar fashion. Usually rapid onset (<48 h). Typical symptoms may be preceded with a prodrome of fever, vomiting, malaise, poor feeding and lethargy which is often indistinguishable from a viral infection. Particularly significant early signs in children include:

• Severe leg pain—so bad that the child can't stand/walk
• Cold hands or feet when the child is running a fever
• Pale skin ± blueness around the lips

Other typical symptoms/signs
Meningism
• Headache
• Photophobia
• Stiff neck—can't put chin on chest
• Kernig's sign +ve—with hips fully flexed resists passive knee extension

↑ Intracranial pressure
• Irritability
• Vomiting
• Drowsiness/↓ consciousness
• ↓ pulse rate
• Fits
• ↑ BP
• Abnormal tone/posturing
• Bulging fontanelle (baby)

Septicaemia/septic shock
• Fever
• Tachypnoea
• Arthritis
• Peripheral shut down—cool peripheries, mottled skin, cyanosis
• Hypotension
• Tachycardia
• ± rash—petechiae suggest meningococcus (Figure 8.3)

⚠ Small children, or immunocompromised patients may not present with typical signs. Go on gut feeling.

⚠ Action
• Call an emergency ambulance and get the patient to hospital as soon as possible.
• If shocked, lie the patient flat and raise legs above waist height
• If symptoms/signs of meningitis or meningococcal septicaemia, give IV/IM benzylpenicillin immediately while awaiting transport. *Dose:*
  • Adult/child ≥10 y—1.2 g
  • Child 1–9 y—600 mg
  • Infant <1 y—300 mg
• Cefotaxime is an alternative for patients allergic to penicillin (adult/child >12 y 1 g; child <12 y 50 mg/kg).
• If possible gain IV access while awaiting the ambulance and take blood for cultures. Consider starting IV fluids/plasma expander. Give 1 l (child—10 ml/kg) rapidly over 10–15 min.
• If available give 100% oxygen.

Contact tracing/prophylaxis for meningococcal meningitis

- Undertaken by the local public health department.
- For a single case only very close contacts ('kissing contacts'), e.g. immediate family members, require prophylactic antibiotics.
- Prophylaxis—rifampicin 600 mg bd for 2 d (child 10 mg/kg bd for 2 d unless <1 y when dose is 5 mg/kg bd for 2 d) or ciprofloxacin 500 mg as a single dose (unlicensed and not suitable for children).
- Rifampicin colours urine red.

❶ Meningitis and acute encephalitis are notifiable diseases.

Telephone helplines for families

Meningitis Research Foundation ☎ 080 8800 3344
🖫 www.meningitis.org.uk
Meningitis Trust ☎ 0800 028 18 28 🖫 www.meningitis-trust.org

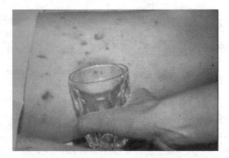

Fig. 8.3 Purpuric rash—does not blanche on pressure with a glass.

☼ Acute stroke

Common and devastating condition—most common cause of adult disability in UK. ½ all strokes occur in people >70 y.

Definitions

- *Stroke:* syndrome typified by rapidly developing signs of focal or global disturbance of cerebral functions, lasting >24 h or leading to death, with no apparent causes other than of vascular origin. (WHO 1978)
- *Transient ischaemic attack (TIA)* or 'mini-stroke': neurological symptoms resolve in <24 h.

Causes

- *Cerebral infarction* (≈70%): atherothrombotic occlusion or embolism. *Sources of embolism:* left atrium (AF) or left ventricle (MI or heart failure). Ischaemia causes direct injury from lack of blood supply.
- *Intracerebral or subarachnoid haemorrhage* (≈ 19%): haemorrhage causes direct neuronal injury and pressure exerted by the blood results in adjacent ischaemia.
- *Rare causes:* sudden ↓BP, vasculitis, venous-sinus thrombosis, carotid artery dissection.

Risk factors

- Age
- ↑BP
- DM
- AF
- Previous stroke or TIA
- Previous MI
- Artificial heart valves
- Hyperviscosity syndromes
- Smoking
- Alcohol
- Obesity
- Low physical activity

Presentation

- *History:* sudden onset of CNS symptoms, or stepwise progression of symptoms over hours or days.
- *Examination:* conscious level may be ↓ or normal; neurological signs (including dysphagia and incontinence); BP; heart rate and rhythm; heart murmurs; carotid bruits; systemic signs of infection or neoplasm.

Differential diagnosis

- Decompensation after recovery from a previous stroke (e.g. due to infection, metabolic disorder)
- Space occupying lesion—1° or 2° cerebral neoplasm, cerebral abscess
- Trauma—subdural haematoma, traumatic brain injury
- Other neurological conditions, e.g. epileptic seizure, migraine, MS.

Acute management

- Admit all patients who have suffered an acute stroke to hospital.
- *Do not* give aspirin prior to admission.
- Recent evidence regarding benefits of thrombolysis means acute admission bypassing the GP altogether will be the norm in future.

Transient ischaemic attack (TIA): presents with a history of sudden onset focal neurological deficit—usually maximal at onset. Recovery takes place within 24 h of initial symptoms. The most common focal deficits are:

• motor symptoms (e.g. hemiparesis or weakness)
• speech or language problems (e.g. dysphagia, dyslexia, or dysarthria)
• sensory symptoms (e.g. visual or somatic sensory symptoms).
   Non-focal symptoms are non-specific and may be due to other causes. They include:

• Light-headedness
• Feeling faint
• Blackouts
• Confusion.

△ Patients with a history of TIA have a 20% risk of stroke in the following month with highest risk in the first 72 h. Risk factors for stroke following TIA are cumulative and include:

• Age ≥60 y
• BP—systolic BP >140 and/or diastolic BP ≥90
• Clinical features—unilateral weakness and/or speech disturbance
• Duration of symptoms ≥10 min (further increased risk if ≥60 min).

Investigations
• ECG
• CXR
• Blood—FBC, ESR, U&E, Cr, lipids, glucose
• Consider clotting screen ± thrombophilia screening if FH thrombosis.

Management of TIA
• Once all symptoms have stopped, start aspirin 50–300 mg od.
• Start treatment for risk factors, e.g. advise to stop smoking, start antihypertensives if ↑ BP.
• Refer for assessment and further investigation to a specialist service, e.g. neurovascular clinic. The National Stroke Guidelines state that all patients with a history of TIA should be seen in a specialist clinic <7 d after the event. Specialist investigations include: CT or MRI scan to confirm diagnosis, carotid dopplers if carotid artery territory symptoms; echocardiogram if recent MI, CCF/LVF or murmur.
• Admit if >1 TIA within 1 wk.

Amaurosis fugax: a form of TIA due to emboli passing through the retina. Causes brief loss of vision (few minutes) 'like a curtain'. Management is as for TIA.

Further information

Royal College of Physicians National clinical guidelines for stroke (2nd edition, 2004) 🖳 www.rcplondon.ac.uk

Cochrane Reviews:
• *Organised inpatient (stroke unit) care for stroke* Stroke Unit Trialists' Collaboration (2002)
• *Thrombolysis for acute ischaemic stroke* Wardlaw et al (2003)

Other neurological emergencies

⌂ **Acute vertigo:** illusion that surroundings are spinning. Ask about previous symptoms and frequency, duration of this attack, nausea/ vomiting, deafness and tinnitus, and recent viral symptoms.

Causes
- *Episodic vertigo lasting a few seconds/minutes:* commonly due to benign positional vertigo.
- *Episodic vertigo lasting minutes to hours:* consider Ménière's (usually associated with hearing loss and tinnitus).
- *Prolonged vertigo (>24 h):* peripheral lesion, e.g. viral labyrinthitis or trauma, or a central lesion (usually associated with other signs), e.g. multiple sclerosis, stroke, tumour.

Examination
- Look for neurological signs especially cerebellar signs and cranial nerve lesions.
- Assess nystagmus, ear drums and hearing.
- Check BP.

Management of acute attacks
- If any signs of ↑ICP (drowsiness, ↓ conscious level, irritability, VI nerve palsy, papilloedema, dropping pulse, rising BP, pupil changes— constriction first then dilatation) or focal neurological signs (except nystagmus), arrange same day neurological opinion or admit depending on the clinical state of the patient.
- If severe symptoms and/or vomiting or significant nausea, treat with a labyrinthine sedative, e.g. cyclizine 50 mg po/IM.
- If mild symptoms, reassure. Symptoms usually settle in <2 wk.

Follow-up: if recurrent attacks or symptoms do not settle, review to further assess the cause of the vertigo.

⊛/⌂**Transverse myelitis:** inflammation of the spinal cord at a single level. Symptoms develop rapidly over days/weeks and include limb weakness, sensory disturbance, bowel and bladder disturbance, back pain and radicular pain. Recovery generally begins in <3 mo but is not always complete.

Causes: idiopathic (thought to be autoimmune mechanism), infection, vaccination, autoimmune disease, e.g. SLE, Sjögren's syndrome, sarcoidosis, MS, malignancy, vascular, e.g. thrombosis of spinal arteries, vasculitis 2° to heroin abuse, spinal A-V malformation.

Management: depending on severity of symptoms, admit as an acute medical emergency or refer for urgent neurological opinion.

☼ **Guillain–Barré polyneuritis:** develops within a few weeks of surgery, 'flu vaccination or infection (URTI, flu, VZ, HSV, cytomegalovirus, EBV, campylobacter; mycoplasma). In 40% no precipitating event is found.

Presentation: ascending motor neuropathy that may advance fast. Proximal muscles are more affected than distal muscles. Trunk, respiratory muscles and cranial nerves are commonly affected.

Management: if suspected admit immediately to hospital as an emergency. Ventilation on ITU is frequently required. 85% make a complete/near complete recovery. *Mortality:* 10%.

⌂ **Ramsay Hunt syndrome (Herpes zoster oticus):** severe pain in the ear precedes facial nerve palsy. Zoster vesicles appear around the ear, in the external ear canal, on the soft palate and in the tonsillar fossa. Often accompanied by deafness ± vertigo, which are slow to resolve and may result in permanent deficit. Pain usually abates after 48 h but postherpetic neuralgia can be a problem. If detected <24 h after the rash appears, treatment with antivirals (e.g. aciclovir 800 mg 5×/d for 1 wk) may be effective.

⌂ **Bell's palsy:** facial palsy without other signs. Unknown cause—possibly viral. *Peak age:* 10–40 y, ♂=♀. *Lifetime incidence:* ~1:65. Affects left and right side of the face equally often.

Presentation: usually sudden onset—may be preceded by pain around the ear. *Other possible symptoms:* facial numbness; ↓ noise tolerance; disturbed taste on the anterior part of the tongue.

Management: ~70% recover completely; 13% have insignificant sequelae; the remainder have permanent deficit. 85% improve in <3 wk—reassure. There is no evidence prednisolone or aciclovir is helpful—results of a large trial are awaited. Protect eye by taping eyelid closed ± protecting the eye with a pad for sleeping, and glasses ± artificial tears if drying in the daytime. *Refer:*
- To neurology or ENT if recovery is not starting after 3 wk
- For tarsorraphy if complete or long-standing palsy
- If unacceptable cosmetic result—may benefit from plastic surgery.

☼ **Brain abscess:** organisms reach the brain via haematogenous spread (primary sites in the heart, lung and bones are most common); direct implantation (trauma, neurosurgery); or local extension from adjacent sites (otitis media, sinusitis, mastoiditis, orbital cellulites). Abscesses can be single or multiple.

Presentation: features usually develop over 2–3 wk (faster if immunosuppressed) and include headache, other features of ↑ICP (drowsiness, ↓ conscious level, irritability, VI nerve palsy, papilloedema, dropping pulse, rising BP, pupil changes—constriction first then dilatation), focal neurological signs—signs depend on where the abscess is, systemic effects of infection (e.g. fever, anorexia, lethargy), and local effects due to cause (e.g. otitis media, new murmur due to SBE).

Management: if suspected, admit as a medical emergency. Treatment is with IV antibiotics ± surgical drainage. Mortality is high (20–30%). 50% of survivors have long-term neurological impairment—30% have epilepsy.

Infections

👁 Infections

Meningitis and encephalitis: 📖 p.148.

Childhood respiratory infections: 📖 p.82.

Acute pneumonia: 📖 p.84.

Influenza: 📖 p.86.

Exacerbations of COPD: 📖 p.88.

Childhood infections: 📖 p.118.

Croup and epiglottitis: 📖 p.76.

Sinusitis: 📖 p.144.

Diarrhoea and vomiting: 📖 p.108.

Eye infections: 📖 p.164.

Urinary tract infection: Childhood – 📖 p.118, Adult – 📖 p.111

Acute otitis externa: causes pain (often severe), discharge from the ear (may be offensive), and hearing loss. If the ear canal is not obscured by debris and discharge, it appears red, swollen and inflamed. Moving the pinna is often painful. There may be associated lymphadenopathy behind or in front of the ear.

Management: prescribe eardrops. Review if persists >1 wk. Options are:
- *Aluminium acetate*—as effective as antibiotic ear drops
- *Antibiotic and/or steroid*—e.g. gentisone HC (contains gentamicin and hydrocortisone)—advise qds administration.

Advise analgesia—OTC paracetamol ± ibuprofen. Consider prescribing stronger analgesia if ineffective.

❶ There is no evidence adding oral antibiotics improves outcome—only use if treatment with drops alone has failed or if administration of ear drops may be difficult and/or less effective, e.g. there is a lot of debris within the canal, the canal is very swollen or the patient is an unco-operative child. Use flucloxacillin or erythromycin 250–500 mg qds. If pseudomonas is suspected use ciprofloxacin (500–750 mg bd)

If there is no response after 1 wk:
- Consider an alternative eardrop, e.g. otosporin (contains neomycin, hydrocortisone and an antifungal—polymyxin B) ± oral antibiotics
- If a swab was taken on initial visit then prescribe based on result
- Consider gentle syringing to remove infected material.

Refer to ENT for aural toilet/advice on further management if there is still no response.

Septic arthritis: most common in children <5 y. Tends to affect hip or knee. The patient is usually systemically unwell and holds the affected joint completely still. Joint may be swollen, hot and tender. Requires emergency admission for IV antibiotics and washout.

Malaria: notifiable disease. 2000 cases/y are notified in the UK.
- *Falciparum malaria:* caused by *Plasmodium falciparum.* Accounts for ~½ UK cases and may not present for up to 3 mo after return from a malarial area. Can be fatal in <24 h—especially if it occurs in small children (<3 y)—cerebral malaria accounts for 80% deaths.
- *Benign malaria:* caused by *P. vivax, P. ovale* and *P. malariae.* May cause illness up to 18 mo after return. All have very low mortality. Relapse may occur at intervals after initial infection as parasites lie dormant in the liver (*P. vivax* and *P. ovale*) or blood (*P. malariae*).

Presentation: easy to miss.
- *Symptoms:* malaria is a great mimic and can present with virtually any symptoms. Usually consists of a prodrome of headache, malaise, myalgia and anorexia followed by recurring high fevers, rigors and drenching sweats—lasting 8–12 h at a time.
- *Examination:* may be normal—look for anaemia, jaundice ± hepatosplenomegaly.

Investigation: in all cases of fever in patients who have returned from a malarial endemic area—even if the plane just landed there and they didn't get off, send a thick and thin film for malaria.

Management: admit for further investigation and treatment if:
- Very unwell—admit without investigation
- Thick and thin film +ve or unable to check thick and thin film (e.g. presentation out of laboratory hours or at a weekend)
- Persistent fever despite -ve thick and thin film.

Wound infection: suspect if a wound becomes painful. Look for swelling, erythema, wound tenderness ± pus. Will usually be treatable in the community unless the patient is systemically unwell.

Management: if pus is present send a swab for M,C&S:
- If the wound is indurated and infection localized to the wound suspect Staphylococcus infection. Treat with flucloxacillin 250–500 mg qds (or erythromycin 250–500 mg qds if penicillin allergy).
- If there is cellulitis around the wound suspect Streptococcus. Treat with penicillin V 250–500 mg qds or erythromycin 250–500 mg qds.
- If foul smelling, suspect anaerobes—use metronidazole 400 mg tds.
Give adequate analgesia; dress the wound frequently; review regularly; allow pus to drain. Refer if simple measures are ineffective.

Prevention of HIV infection in exposed individuals
- Refer to A&E for prophylaxis if inadvertent exposure through needle stick injury or similar.
- Consider prophylaxis if sexual contact with an infected (or high risk if status unknown) individual <72 h before presentation—take advice from GUM clinic.

Eye emergencies

⊛ Assessment of eye emergencies

History: most patients attend with symptoms of visual loss, pain in or around the eye, or changed appearance of the eye. *Points to cover:*

Is there any visual loss? If there is:
- Was the visual loss sudden or gradual?
- Was it associated with distortion of the visual image? Distinguish between blurred and double vision.
- Was distance, near vision, colour or peripheral vision affected first?
- Was it associated with pain in the eye or was it painless?

Consider:
- Eye disease
- Drugs
- CNS lesions
  - *Visual field loss*—vascular lesions, e.g. stroke
  - *Double vision*—MS, trauma, tumour, basilar artery insufficiency, chronic basilar meningitis
  - *Flashing lights*—migraine, seizure
  - *Visual hallucinations*—seizure, drugs
  - *Transient blindness*—vascular lesions, migraine

Is there any eye pain? If there is:
- Is the eye gritty or aching?
- Is it associated with photophobia or headache?

Consider:
- *Painful conditions:* corneal abrasion, foreign body, keratitis, iritis, scleritis, acute glaucoma, ophthalmic shingles, arc eye.
- *Eye discomfort:* conjunctivitis, entropion, trichasis, dry eye, episcleritis, optic neuritis.
- *Referred pain:* tension type headache, migraine, refractive error, trigeminal neuralgia (📖 p.146), ophthalmic shingles, giant cell arteritis (📖 p.146), ocular muscle imbalance, raised intracranial pressure.

Is there any change in appearance of the eye? Ask about redness, discharge, or other change in appearance of the eye.

Other points to cover
- Has there been any eye trauma?
- Have there been any previous, similar episodes?
- Does the patient or any other family member suffer from any systemic illness?
- Is there any eye disease in the family?

Examination: use a systematic approach. Consider:
- The external eye
- The ocular media
- Visual acuity
- Visual fields
- Eye movements
- Pupils

Table 10.1 Eye referrals

Emergency referral (direct to A&E or emergency eye clinic)	Sudden loss of vision—📖 p.170
	Acute glaucoma—📖 p.172
	Perforating injury—📖 p.175
	Intraocular foreign body—📖 p.175
	Blunt injury with hyphema—📖 p.174
	Chemical burns—📖 p.175
	Retinal detachment—📖 p.171
	Corneal ulcer—📖 p.166
	Sudden onset of diplopia or squint + pain
	Temporal arteritis with visual symptoms—📖 p.146
Urgent (within 12 h)	Vitreous haemorrhage—📖 p.170
	Orbital fracture—📖 p.174
	Sudden onset of ocular inflammation, e.g. iritis or ophthalmic herpes zoster/simplex—📖 p.166–168
	Corneal foreign bodies or abrasions—📖 p.174
Soon (within 1–2 wk)	Central visual loss
	Sinister 'floaters'—📖 p.171
	Flashing lights without a field defect—📖 p.171
	Chronic glaucoma with pressure >30 mmHg
Routine referral	Gradual loss of vision
	Chronic glaucoma (pressure <30 mmHg)
	Chronic red eye conditions
	Painless diplopia or squint
	Chalazion/stye/cyst
	Ptosis
	Headaches and migraine*—📖 p.142
	Chronic watery eye

*Urgent if sinister cause suspected.

❶ Community-based optometrists, with their experience, equipment and training are a valuable resource available to GPs to help differentiate eye conditions and refine referral pathways. Getting an optometrist's opinion can also assist in setting the appropriate priority level for referral or prevent unnecessary referrals.

External eye

- The eyelids should be symmetrical—drooping or elevation of the upper lid may be due to nerve lesions or thyroid disease.
- Check the skin around the lids, the eyelash position, and any inflammation, crusting or swelling of the lid or lid margin.
- Then examine the eye surface—it should be bright and shiny. Use a fluorescein stain if any indication of corneal damage. Note any redness—if most marked around the lid lining and periphery of the eye conjunctivitis is likely, where as a duskier redness around the margin of the cornea (ciliary congestion) suggests disease of the cornea, iris or deeper parts of the eye (uvea).

Examining the ocular media: takes practice. Darken the room and ensure you have good batteries in the ophthalmoscope.
- Check the red reflex (opacities within the eye appear as a shadow).
- Then focus on to the retina—use a systematic approach to avoid missing anything—i.e. start at the optic disc (look for shape, colour and size of the cup) and then follow each of the 4 main vessels to the periphery.
- End by examining the macula: ask the patient to look directly at the light.
- Dilating the pupils with a short-acting mydriatic (e.g. 0.5–1% tropicamide) makes examination much easier—warn patients they may have temporarily blurred vision and should not drive.

Visual acuity: test and record the central (macular) vision of each eye separately (with glasses on if worn) for both near and distance. Cover the non-test eye carefully. On a full size Snellen chart, line '6' can be read by the normal eye at 6 m. Near vision can be checked using a newspaper or a near vision testing card (see opposite). If patients have forgotten their glasses use a 'pin hole' to look through (it removes most refractive problems).

Visual fields: test peripheral vision by sitting in front of the patient and comparing their visual field to your own (one eye at a time)—the most basic test is to check the patient can see hand movement in each of the four quadrants. This may reveal hemianopia from damage to visual pathways or field loss due to glaucoma (the patient may be unaware of the loss). Refer for formal tests if necessary.

Eye movements: if the patient complains of double vision, move an object to the 6 positions of gaze—upper, middle and lower right, follow the object across to the opposite side and then upper, middle and lower left ('H' shaped movement)—to check when the double vision occurs.

Pupils: should be round, central and of equal size. They should respond equally to light and accommodation.

N.48

She waved

N.36

Faces the sun

N.24

Painting the rainbow

N.18

Life was like a flying dogfish

N.14

Quietly a storm drove purple ducks
across the road. The chimney top

N.12

Glowed in the dusk and my sister let her
biscuit fall through ashes. September was

N.10

In drizzling mood when hedgehogs threw pinecones
in the dark. Squirrels played classical music.

N.8

We won a feather duster by encouraging Jessica to bake an
enormous apple pie and pirouette between the tables.

N.6

Queuing had never appealed to the young porcupines but swimming held great drama
for the blue and pink ostrich.

N.5

Delight was exceeding the pleasures of everyday ambulation and breaking the pattern of a melancholy
existence to see the trees.

The red eye

> ⚠ **'Red flag' signs of a potentially dangerous red eye**
> - ↓ visual acuity
> - Pain deep in the eye—not surface irritation as with conjunctivitis
> - Absent or sluggish pupil response
> - Corneal damage on fluorescein staining
> - History of trauma.
>
> Refer the patient to be seen by a specialist the same day. Have a lower threshold to refer if recently post-op.

⊛ **Conjunctivitis:** inflammation of the conjunctiva is the commonest eye problem seen in general practice—1:8 children have an episode of acute infective conjunctivitis every year.

Presentation: red, sore eye (Figure 10.1), eye discharge—clear, mucoid or mucopurulent, sticking of the eyelids—especially on waking. No change in visual acuity. Examination may reveal enlarged papillae under the upper eyelid and/or pre-auricular lymph node enlargement.

Bacterial or viral conjunctivitis: clinically difficult to distinguish. Both present with acute red eye—usually starting in one eye and often spreading to involve both, together with watery/purulent discharge. The eyes are often crusted ± stuck together on waking. Visual acuity is not impaired. Both may occur in association with viral URTI.

Management
- Recent evidence shows that in ~85% of cases, acute infective conjunctivitis clears in <7 d with or without treatment.
- Advise patients to bathe the affected eye(s) with boiled, cooled water morning and night.
- If symptoms are not improving in >5 d, take a swab for M,C&S (± Chlamydia) and treat empirically with chloramphenicol qds or fucithalmic bd for 5 d. ❶ Chloramphenicol eye drops are available over-the-counter.
- If still not clearing, then act on swab results or consider alternative diagnosis, e.g. allergy, dry eyes.

⚠ Advise patients to see a doctor if: ↓ visual acuity, eye becomes painful rather than sore/gritty, or symptoms are not improving in 5 d.

Ophthalmia neonatorum: caused by *N. gonorrhoea.* Presents as a purulent discharge from the eyes of an infant <21 d old. Send swabs for M,C&S. Treat with hourly ofloxacin eye drops. Refer for urgent ophthalmology opinion as cornea may perforate.

Allergic conjunctivitis: bilateral symptoms appear seasonally (e.g. hay fever) or on contact with an allergen (e.g. animal fur). Presents with red, watery, itchy eyes ± photophobia ± family or personal history of atopy. *Examination:* follicles in the lower tarsal conjunctiva and 'cobblestones' under the upper lid.

Management: Treat with topical or systemic antihistamines (e.g. sodium cromoglycate eye drops, loratidine). Avoid topical steroids due to long-term complications (cataract, glaucoma, fungal infection). Refer if persistent.

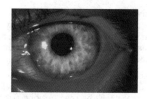

Fig. 10.1 Acute conjunctivitis.

Table 10.2 Differential diagnosis of red eye

Structure	Condition
Inflammation of the orbit	Thyroid eye disease/exomphalos
	Orbital cellulitis (📖 p.166)
	Tumour
Lid disease	Stye/chalazion
	Blepharitis
	Allergic eye disease
Scleral inflammation	Scleritis/episcleritis (📖 p.168)
	Postoperative inflammation
Conjunctival disease	Infection (viral, bacterial or chlamydial—opposite)
	Allergy (opposite)
	Subconjunctival haemorrhage (📖 p.166)
Corneal disease	Foreign body/trauma (📖 p.174)
	Corneal abrasion (📖 p.174)
	Dry eye syndrome
	Ophthalmic shingles (📖 p.168)
	Corneal ulceration (📖 p.166)
	Arc eye (📖 p.175)
Uveal/iris inflammation	Anterior uveitis (📖 p.168)
	Posterior uveitis/toxoplasma
Other causes of red eye	Acute glaucoma (📖 p.172)
	Postoperative endophthalmitis

⊙ **Subconjunctival haemorrhage:** spontaneous painless localized haemorrhage under the conjunctiva (Figure 10.2). Common in the elderly. Looks alarming but generally painless (may cause some aching of the eye). Clears spontaneously in 1–2 wk but may recur. *Associations:* ↑BP, clotting disorders, leukaemia, ↑ venous pressure.

Management: Check BP. If severe/recurrent, check FBC and clotting screen. Consider referral if follows trauma—especially if the posterior edge of the haemorrhage can't be seen (may be associated with orbital haematoma, penetrating injury or orbital fracture).

⊛ **Orbital cellulitis:** typically due to spread of infection from the paranasal sinuses. Usually presents with pain, double/blurred vision, and general malaise. *Signs:* fever, eyelid swelling, proptosis and inability to move the eye. Severe cases can lead to septicaemia, meningitis and cavernous sinus thrombosis. If suspected, refer immediately to ophthalmology for IV antibiotics/surgical drainage.

Preseptal cellulitis: infections of the upper lid may cause significant swelling and redness around the eye. Typically affects children following mild trauma. The eye is unaffected—infection is localized to skin and superficial tissues. Treat as localized cellulitis with oral antibiotics (e.g. flucloxacillin). Monitor carefully as can progress to orbital cellulitis.

◬ **Keratitis, keratoconjunctivitis and corneal ulceration**
- Keratitis is inflammation of the cornea
- Keratoconjunctivitis is inflammation of the conjunctiva and cornea.

Presentation: very painful eye, blurred vision, photophobia and profuse watering. On examination there is ↓ visual acuity, circumcorneal injection (blood vessel dilatation concentrated around the limbus), conjunctivitis (particularly the quadrant most associated with the injury/infection) ± a creamy white, disc-shaped lesion on the central or inferior cornea (corneal ulcer—Figure 10.3). The pupil may be small due to reflex miosis. Corneal ulcers stain green with fluorescein—use a bright light with a blue filter to see them.

Causes
- Bacterial—2° to trauma, foreign body, dry eyes, entropion, blepharitis
- Viral—herpes simplex, herpes zoster or adenovirus
- Fungal
- Protozoal—history of foreign travel/contact lens wear
- Non-infective, e.g. 2° to autoimmune disease or trauma.

Management: treatment depends on cause. Delay in treatment may result in loss of sight so refer for same-day ophthalmology assessment.

Herpes simplex infection: common and can be recurrent in the same eye. Presents with acute keratitis/kerato-conjunctivitis. Examination and fluorescein staining reveal a characteristic corneal ulcer (dendritic ulcer)—Figure 10.4. Always refer for urgent (same-day) ophthalmology opinion. Treatment is with 3% aciclovir ointment 5×/d continued for 3 d after healing.

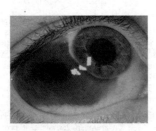

Fig. 10.2 Subconjunctival haemorrhage.

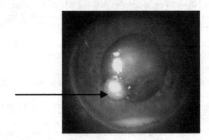

Fig. 10.3 Corneal ulcer.

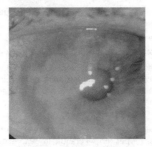

Fig. 10.4 Dendritic ulcer.

⚠ There is a danger of massive amoebic ulceration and blindness if steroid eye drops are administered to patients with dendritic ulcer.

⚱ **Ophthalmic shingles:** zoster in the ophthalmic branch of the oculomotor (IIIrd) nerve. Pain, tingling or numbness around the eye precedes a blistering rash and inflammation. In 50% the eye is affected with conjunctivitis, scleritis, episcleritis, keratitis, iritis, visual loss and/or occulomotor nerve palsy. Nose tip involvement makes eye involvement likely (nerve supply is the same as the globe)—Figure 10.5. Prescribe oral aciclovir (800 mg 5×/d) and refer immediately. The cornea may become anaesthetic/scarred and require grafting.

⚱ **Epislceritis:** the episclera is the thin layer of vascular tissue overlying the sclera. Episcleritis is unilateral in 2:3 cases. It presents with diffuse inflammation of the eye with minimal tenderness and no discharge. Try treatment with an NSAID (e.g. ibuprofen 400 mg tds or ketorolac 0.5% eye drops qds). If a NSAID is ineffective, refer to ophthalmology for consideration of treatment with steroids.

⚱ **Scleritis:** inflammation of the sclera. Can be unilateral or bilateral. ♀>♂. Peak age: 40–60 y. Affects the anterior or posterior segment and may be diffuse, nodular or necrotizing.

Presentation: painful, red eye. Vision may be blurred due to corneal, iris or posterior segment involvement, and visual acuity ↓. The eye is tender to touch, and may have a deep purple hue. Look for scleral nodules. There may be accompanying uveitis and keratitis.

Associations: in ~50%, associated with systemic illness, e.g. herpes zoster, rheumatoid arthritis, systemic lupus erythematosus, polyarteritis nodosum, Wegener's granulomatosis, trauma, infection, or surgery.

Management: refer urgently to ophthalmology for confirmation of diagnosis and specialist management with steroids. Complications include cataract, glaucoma, and retinal detachment.

⚱ **Iritis (anterior uveitis):** most common in young/middle-aged adults.

Presentation: acute onset of pain, photophobia, blurred vision and ↓ visual acuity, watering, circum-corneal redness, small or irregular pupil ± keratitic precipitates on the posterior surface of the cornea (Figure 10.6) ± hypopyon (anterior chamber pus, causing a white 'fluid-level' line). Pain ↑ as eyes converge and pupils constrict.

Causes: may be secondary to corneal graft rejection or eye infections, e.g. toxoplasmosis, herpes virus keratitis. In 30% associated with seronegative arthropathies, e.g. ankylosing spondylitis.

Management: refer urgently to ophthalmology for confirmation of diagnosis and specialist management. Complications include posterior synechiae (irregular pupil shape), glaucoma and cataract. Relapses are common.

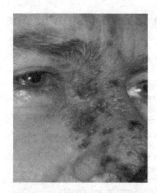

Fig. 10.5 Ophthalmic shingles.

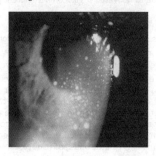

Fig. 10.6 Keratic precipitates in a patient with anterior uveitis.

⚠ Sudden loss of vision in one eye

⚠ Always refer as an emergency to ophthalmology (unless you are sure it is migraine or stroke)

Causes of sudden loss of vision covered elsewhere
- Migraine (📖 p.144)
- Stroke/amaurosis fugax (📖 p.150)
- Temporal arteritis (📖 p.146).

Retinal vein occlusion: incidence ↑ with age. More common than arterial occlusion. Presents with:
- Sudden loss of vision in 1 eye—typically on waking (branch retinal vein occlusion causes partial visual loss).
- Fundus like 'a stormy sunset'—scattered haemorrhages, engorged veins, disc swelling ± cotton wool spots
- ± painful eye due to neovascular glaucoma ± afferent pupil defect.

Causes
- Glaucoma
- Arteriosclerosis
- ↑BP
- Polycythaemia
- Hypercholesterolaemia
- ↑ homocysteine

Management: refer as an emergency to ophthalmology.

Retinal artery occlusion: usually due to thrombo-embolism. Presents with sudden visual loss in 1 eye (counting fingers or light perception) and afferent pupil defect. The retina appears white ± cherry red spot at the macular. A retinal embolus may be visible. Exclude temporal arteritis (📖 p.146). Refer as an emergency to ophthalmology for confirmation of diagnosis. Treat any risk factors for atherosclerosis or embolism, i.e. ↑BP, hyperlipidaemia, smoking, DM, carotid/cardiac disease.

⚠ **If the patient presents <1 h after onset:** applying then releasing firm eyeball pressure can sometimes dislodge an embolus into one of the smaller branches and thus preserve some vision.

Anterior ischaemic optic neuropathy (ANION): occurs when the short ciliary arteries are damaged. 2 forms:
- *Arteritic:* due to arterial inflammation (e.g. temporal arteritis, SLE)
- *Non-arteritic:* results from arterial emboli.

Presentation and management: central vision drops suddenly and irreversibly. Examination reveals a complete or altitudinal visual field defect. The disc appears swollen and pale ± haemorrhages. May be accompanied by symptoms of the underlying condition (e.g. temporal arteritis—📖 p.146). Refer as an ophthalmology emergency. Treatment depends on cause.

Vitreous haemorrhage: presents with sudden ↓ in vision, loss of red reflex, and difficulty visualizing the retina. *Risk factors:* DM with new vessel formation, bleeding disorders, retinal tear/detachment, central retinal vein occlusion, trauma, head injury, tumour. Refer urgently to ophthalmology for confirmation of diagnosis and treatment.

Retinal detachment: affects 1:5000 people each year. Presents with:
- Painless loss of vision—'like a curtain' coming across the vision.
- Rate of detachment can vary. Upper retinal detachments tend to occur more quickly—causing loss of lower part of vision.
- 50% have premonitory symptoms—flashing lights or spots before eyes due to abnormal retinal stimulation prior to the detachment.
- If the macular is detached (more common in upper detachments) central vision is lost and does not completely recover—even after retinal reattachment.
- Examination reveals visual field loss (± central visual loss), afferent pupil defect and a grey retina that may balloon forwards.

Causes
- Idiopathic
- Trauma
- DM (fibrous bands in the vitreous)
- After cataract surgery
- Myopia
- Retinopathy of prematurity
- Inherited eye disease

Management: refer urgently to ophthalmology for treatment to secure the retina.

Floaters: small dark spots in the visual field usually caused by opacities in the vitreous. Floaters continue to move when the eye comes to rest. *Risk factors:* myopia, cataract operation, trauma. Usually harmless and may settle with time.

⚠ Sudden showers of floaters in 1 eye ± flashing lights can indicate retinal detachment which may be difficult to see on examination. Floaters associated with eye pain/inflammation may indicate posterior uveitis.

General rules for referral
- If long-standing floaters/flashes then no need for referral
- If symptoms are of recent onset (<6 wk) and no other symptoms, refer urgently to ophthalmology out-patients
- If symptoms are of recent onset (<6 wk) and associated with any visual field loss, ↓ acuity, or pain/inflammation of the eye, refer as an ophthalmology emergency.

Optic neuritis: disc swelling due to inflammation or demyelination. Presents with:
- Rapid visual loss (hours–days) and ↓ colour vision (red desaturation)
- Discomfort on eye movements
- Temporary worsening of symptoms when hot
- Optic disc swelling.

Causes: MS (1:4 patients with MS present with optic neuritis); DM; viral infections, e.g. influenza, measles, chickenpox; familial, e.g. Leber's disease.

Management: refer urgently to ophthalmology for confirmation of diagnosis. Steroids may help in severe cases. Visual loss usually stabilizes after week 2 and recovers over 6 wk.

Acute closed-angle glaucoma (AACG): uncommon, Affects 0.1% of patients >40 y—typically elderly, long-sighted women with early cataract.

Presentation
- *Latent:* usually picked up when screening the opposite eye after an episode of acute or subacute glaucoma. The patient is asymptomatic and intraocular pressure is normal but the eye has a shallow anterior chamber with narrow angle.
- *Subacute:* episodic haloes around bright lights, impaired vision ± frontal headache/eye pain. Attacks are precipitated by the pupil dilating, e.g. at night or when entering a darkened room and relieved by sleep or entering a brighter environment. Examination between attacks is normal but during an attack, the pupil is semi-dilated and cornea slightly clouded. Patients with subacute glaucoma are at risk of an acute attack.
- *Acute:* blockage of aqueous drainage from the anterior chamber causes a sudden ↑2° in intra-ocular pressure from 15–20 to 60–70 mmHg. There may be a history of previous subacute attacks. The patient complains of eye pain with acute loss of vision in one eye ± abdominal pain/nausea/vomiting.

Examination: vision ↓; cornea looks hazy (due to oedema); pupil is fixed and dilated (often slightly oval in shape with long axis vertical); circum-corneal redness; eyeball feels hard (due to ↑ pressure); poor fundal view ± cataract.

Tip for detection of acute glaucoma:
- Shine a light sideways across the eye (from the outer angle of the eye straight across directly towards the nose)
- In the normal eye the iris is lit up
- In the eye with AACG, the central part of the iris remains shaded.

Management: refer acute or subacute glaucoma as an emergency to ophthalmology

Follow-up: AACG may damage the trabecular meshwork and patients are at risk of developing chronic glaucoma following an attack. Regular check-ups are necessary.

Wet (neovascular) age-related macular degeneration: always a bilateral disease, but 1 eye is usually more severely affected than the other. Subretinal blood vessel formation (choroidal neovascularization). causes rapidly progressive distortion of vision and central visual loss. Eventually a dense scar forms and the patient sees a dense black patch in the centre of vision but is able to use peripheral vision to navigate/see in the distance.

Risk factors: ↑ age, +ve family history, smoking, ↑BP.

Presentation
- Deterioration/distortion of central vision—affects reading/face recognition first—worse with changes in lighting.
- A dark patch that rapidly fades may be noticed on waking—can be interpreted as 'seeing a shadowy figure' and be very frightening.
- With severe visual loss patients may see visual hallucinations—usually of faces or stars. These can also be very frightening.

Examination: ↓ acuity; afferent pupil defect with severe visual loss; decompensated squint. Look for macular drusen (yellow/white subretinal spots); pigment and sub-retinal haemorrhage ± oedema. The disc should look normal.

Management: refer for urgent retinal opinion if recent onset of visual loss. Most visual loss occurs within the first 2 mo. Laser photocoagulation and photodynamic therapy can help some patients with the rapidly progressive neovascular form.

Eye trauma

⊚ Corneal abrasions

- Take a careful history to exclude high-speed particles (e.g. from strimmer etc.) that could cause penetrating injury.
- Abrasions may cause severe pain—if so apply a few drops of local anaesthetic (e.g. oxybuprocaine 0.4%) before examining. Use fluorescein stain, with blue light illumination to detect abrasion (Figure 10.7).
- If the abrasion is vertical, ensure no foreign body is left in the eye by everting the upper lid.
- Abrasions normally heal in <48 h.
- Prescribe chloramphenicol drops qds until healing is complete.
- Eye padding is not needed except to protect the eye after a local anaesthetic.

⊚ Superficial foreign bodies: cause discomfort, a 'foreign body sensation' and watering. They can be difficult to see so examine very carefully (Figure 10.8), including everting the eyelids. The foreign body sensation may come from an abrasion.

Management

- If metal or a penetrating injury is suspected, refer to eye casualty.
- Superficial foreign bodies can be removed with a corner of clean card after instilling local anaesthetic. If that fails, you can try using the tip of a sterile green needle (bent if necessary)—but be careful. Refer to eye casualty if you are not confident.
- After removal, treat with topical antibiotics, e.g. chloramphenicol 2-hourly for 3 d then qds for 5 d.
- If left >12 h, a rust ring may form around a metal foreign body—refer to eye casualty for removal.

⌂ Blunt injury: caused by fists, squash balls, etc. The result may be anything from a 'black eye' to globe rupture. Globe rupture is usually obvious with a wound and severely ↓ vision. More minor injuries include subconjunctival haemorrhage or corneal abrasion.

Urgently refer if:

- Visual acuity is affected or double vision
- Lacerated conjunctiva or hyphaema—blood in the anterior chamber
- Unable to see posterior limit of a subconjunctival haemorrhage—may indicate orbital fracture
- Persistent pupil dilation—usually recovers spontaneously but may indicate a torn iris
- Any signs of retinal damage (oedema, choroidal rupture), or
- If you cannot assess the eye, e.g. due to lid swelling or pain.

⌂ 'Blow out' fracture of the orbit: uncommon fracture due to blunt trauma to the eye (e.g. squash ball injury). Signs include enophthalmos (often masked by swelling), infraorbital nerve loss and inability to look upwards due to trapping of inferior rectus muscle. Refer for X-ray and assessment of eye trauma via A&E.

⊛/⊿ **Penetrating wounds:** refer urgently to eye casualty if penetrating injury is a possibility, i.e. history of flying object or working with hammers, drills, lathes or chisels where a metal fragment may fly off. X-ray/CT Scan can confirm diagnosis and help locate the foreign body.

Symptoms/signs: ❶ Wound may be tiny
- Vision may initially be normal, or may be very poor, depending on the size of the foreign body.
- Eye is painful and waters
- Look for photophobia, hyphaema (blood in anterior chamber) and/or pupil distortion.

⚠ *Do not remove large foreign bodies (dart or knife)*—support the object with padding while transferring the patient supine to eye casualty or A&E. Cover the other eye to prevent damage from conjugate movement.

⊿ **Chemical burns:** can cause great damage—particularly alkali injuries. Use topical anaesthetic (e.g. oxybuprocaine 0.4%) before examining. Hold the lids open, brush out any powder and irrigate with large amounts (1–2 l) of clean saline or water immediately. Don't try to neutralize the acid or alkali. Refer urgently to eye casualty.

⊛ **Arc eye:** due to corneal epithelial damage as a result of exposure to UV light. Seen in welders, sunbed users, skiers, mountaineers and sailors who don't use adequate eye protection. Symptoms include severe eye pain, watering and blepharospasm a few hours after exposure.

Management: pad the eye and give analgesics and cyclopentolate 1% eye drops bd (causes pupil dilation). Recovery should occur in <24 h—if not refer. Advise on suitable protective wear for future exposure.

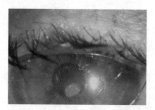

Fig. 10.7 Corneal abrasion: Stained with fluorescein appears green.

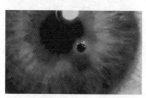

Fig. 10.8 Corneal foreign body.

Endocrine emergencies

☼ Endocrine emergencies

Hypoglycaemia: known diabetic on oral/insulin therapy. Short history. May present with coma, fits or odd/violent behaviour, tachycardia ± ↑ BP. There may or may not have been warning signs/symptoms—sweating, hunger, tremor. ❶ Younger children may present atypically with behavioural changes or headache.

Investigation: blood sugar (on blood testing strip) <2.5 mmol/l.

> ⚠ *Action*
> - If conscious give simple carbohydrate, e.g. 3 glucose tablets, 100 ml of a sugar-containing soft drink, e.g. Lucozade®, or Hypostop®
> - If unable to take oral carbohydrate—give IM glucagon 1 mg IM (children <25 kg–0.5 mg)—takes ≤5 min to act—may have poor effect if the patient is starved or drunk—*or* IV glucose (*adult:* 50–250 ml of 10% solution in 50 ml aliquots; *child:* 2–5 ml/kg of 10% solution)
> - Once the patient has regained consciousness supplement with simple carbohydrate as for the conscious patient and as symptoms improve give complex carbohydrate, e.g. biscuits
> - Repeat glucose testing in <15 min then monitor frequent blood sugars over the next 4 h (hourly) and 4-hourly for the following 24 h
> - Maintain a high glucose intake for several hours if the patient has a severe episode of hypoglycaemia due to a sulphonylurea
> - Review reasons for the hypoglycaemia.

Hyperglycaemic ketoacidotic coma: only occurs in patients with type 1 DM though may be the way in which it presents (i.e. can occur in young patients not known to be diabetic). Presents with a 2–3 d history of deterioration often precipitated by infection. Typically the patient is dehydrated with Kussmaul breathing (deep sighing breaths), ketotic (fruity) smelling breath, shock (↓ BP and postural drop, tachycardia) ± coma. ⚠ Can present with vomiting and abdominal pain mimicking acute abdomen—always check for ketotic breath and Kussmaul breathing.

Investigation: BM is usually >20 mmol/l and urine (if available) tests +ve for ketones.

> ⚠ *Action*
> Arrange to admit as an emergency to hospital. If shocked/coma—lie flat, elevate feet and resuscitate:
> - Airway—check airway is clear
> - Breathing—give 100% O₂ if available
> - Circulation—gain IV access if possible and give 1 l (child: 10 ml/kg) 0.9% saline rapidly. Repeat up to 3× as needed.

Hyperglycaemic hyperosmolar non-ketotic coma: only occurs in patients with type 2 DM. Presents with <1 wk history of deterioration, ↓ level of consciousness, dehydration ++, ↓ BP with postural drop. Often precipitated by other illness, e.g. infection, MI. May be a presenting feature of type 2 DM. Blood sugar (on blood testing strip) >35 mmol/l.

> ⚠ *Action:* admit immediately to hospital.

Myxoedema coma
Presentation
- >65 y old
- History of thyroid surgery/radioactive iodine
- May be precipitated by MI, stroke, infection or trauma
- Looks hypothyroid
- Hypothermia
- Hyporeflexia
- Heart failure
- Cyanosis
- Bradycardia
- Coma
- Seizures

Investigation: finger prick blood glucose may be ↓.

⚠ **Action**
- Keep warm
- Treat heart failure with diuretics ± opioids and nitrates—📖 p.78
- Admit as an emergency to hospital.

Hyperthyroid crisis (thyrotoxic storm)
Risk factors
- Recent thyroid surgery/radioactive iodine
- Infection
- Trauma
- MI

Presentation
- Fever
- Agitation and/or confusion
- Coma
- Tachycardia/AF
- Diarrhoea and vomiting
- Acute abdomen
- May have goitre ± thyroid bruit.

⚠ **Action:** admit as an emergency to hospital.

Hypoadrenal (Addisonian) crisis: may occur in patients on long-term steroids (treatment or replacement) if the steroids are stopped suddenly or not ↑ during intercurrent illness, *or* may be a presenting feature of congenital adrenal hyperplasia or Addison's disease. Presents with vomiting, hypotension and shock.

Management: give IM or IV hydrocortisone:
- Adults and children >12 y: 100 mg
- Children 1 mo–12y: 2–4 mg/kg

Admit to hospital for further management.

Prevention of Addisonian crises
- Warn all patients taking long-term steroids not to stop their steroids abruptly and to tell any doctor treating them about their condition.
- Advise patients to carry a steroid card or Addison's disease self-help group emergency card, and wear a medicalert bracelet or similar in case of emergency.
- Double dose of steroid prior to dental treatment or if intercurrent illness (e.g. URTI).
- If vomiting, replace oral steroid with IM hydrocortisone.

Gynaecological and obstetric emergencies

Acute gynaecological problems

Acute pelvic pain: causes—Table 12.1.

History: ask about:
• Timing and quality of pain
• Precipitating and relieving factors
• Relationship to menstrual cycle (and possibility of pregnancy)
• Dyspareunia
• Bowel and bladder symptoms
• History of ectopic pregnancy
• Pelvic infection or surgery
• Psychological problems.

Examination and investigation
• Abdominal examination—including rectal examination
• Pelvic and vaginal examination—normal pelvic and vaginal examination, if adequate examination is possible, makes a gynaecological cause unlikely
• Pregnancy test if appropriate.

Management: admit unless cause is known and ectopic pregnancy (📖 p.188) can be excluded.

Acute pelvic inflammatory disease (PID): only 70% of those with acute PID clinically, have diagnosis confirmed on laparoscopy. Most cases are associated with sexually transmitted infections. In 20% no cause is found. Usual organisms are Chlamydia (50%) and/or Gonorrhoea.

History
• Fever >38°C and malaise
• Acute pelvic pain (usually bilateral) and deep dyspareunia
• Dysuria
• Abnormal vaginal bleeding— heavier periods, intermenstrual and/or postcoital bleeding
• Purulent vaginal discharge

Examination
• Pyrexia
• Vaginal discharge
• Cervical excitation
• Adnexal tenderness

Investigations: consider
• *Swabs*—high vaginal swab and endocervical swab for M,C&S and chlamydia screening
• *Blood*—FBC—may show leucocytosis, ↑ ESR/CRP.

Management: admit if very unwell or ectopic pregnancy or other acute surgical emergency cannot be excluded, otherwise:
• Advise rest and sexual abstinence, provide analgesia
• Treat with ofloxacin 400 mg bd and metronidazole 400 mg bd for 14 d. If the patient has an IUCD consider removal but only if symptoms are severe. If removed advise re alternative contraception and emergency contraception if sexual intercourse <7 d ago.
• Arrange contact tracing via GUM clinic
• If no improvement after 48 h admit; if slow recovery consider referral for laparoscopy to exclude abscess formation.

Severe dysmenorrhoea: lower abdominal cramps ± backache occuring in the first 1–2 d of a period. May be associated GI disturbance, e.g. diarrhoea/vomiting. Treat with NSAID, e.g. mefenamic acid (500 mg tds), naproxen (500 mg initially then 250 mg 6–8 hourly), ibuprofen (200–400 mg tds)—effective in 80–90%.

Ovarian hyperstimulation: iatrogenic condition resulting from overstimulation of the ovaries in the course of infertility treatment.

- *Mild hyperstimulation:* >10% patients receiving gonadotrophin therapy. Ovaries enlarge and cysts form resulting in abdominal pain and swelling ± vomiting/diarrhoea. Manage with rest and simple analgesia, e.g. ibuprofen or paracetamol prn.
- *Severe hyperstimulation:* 1% patients receiving gonadotrophin therapy. Abdominal pain/distention, vomiting/diarrhoea, ascites, pleural effusion, and/or venous thrombosis. Admit.

Cervical shock: rare complication of intrauterine device (IUCD) insertion. Presents with pallor, sweating, and bradycardia. Immediately tip the woman head down with legs raised. If symptoms/bradycardia persist, give 0.6 mg atropine IV.

⚠ **Women with epilepsy:** ↑ risk of seizure at the time of cervical dilation—ensure emergency drugs are available.

Very heavy menstrual bleeding

- Resuscitate as necessary—admit if shocked—D&C in the acute situation can ↓ haemorrhage by 75–80%
- Correct anaemia
- Stop bleeding with progestogen, e.g. norethisterone 5 mg tds for 10 d. Effective in 24–48 h. A lighter bleed will follow on stopping. Alternatively consider tranexamic acid (1 g tds for 4 d) to ↓ bleeding
- Refer for gynaecology assessment.

Table 12.1 Causes of pelvic pain

Gynaecological		Non-gynaecological	
Acute	**Chronic**	**Acute**	**Chronic**
Ectopic pregnancy	Endometriosis	Appendicitis	Irritable bowel syndrome
Infection	Adhesions	Cystitis	
Endometriosis	Fibroids	Neurological	Musculoskeletal
Torsion of fibroid	Ovarian cyst	Colitis	Psychological
Dysmenorrhoea	Venous congestion	Psychological	Bowel or bladder cancer
Ovarian cyst (torsion, bleeding or rupture)	Pelvic inflammatory disease		Neurological

Further information

RCOG Management of acute pelvic inflammatory disease (2003) ▣ www.rcog.org.uk
British Association for Sexual Health and HIV (BASHH) Management of PID (2005) ▣ www.bashh.org

👁 Emergency contraception

History: ask:
- when the woman's last menstrual period started and usual cycle length
- when she had unprotected intercourse and whether there were other episodes of unprotected intercourse during this cycle
- what other medication she is taking, including contraceptive pills
- whether she has any chronic or current medical conditions,

Hormonal emergency contraception: *BNF 7.3.1.* Use levo-norgestrel 1.5 mg—available OTC and on prescription. Single dose taken <72 h (3 d) after unprotected intercourse—the sooner it is taken, the greater the efficacy:
- 0–24 h—95% efficacy
- 25–48 h—85% efficacy
- 49–72 h—58% efficacy

❶ Levonorgestrel is effective up to 120 h post-intercourse (unlicensed >3 d) but effectiveness ↓ the longer the delay.

Contraindications: acute active porphyria, severe liver disease, allergy.

Possible pitfalls
- *Vomiting <3 h after taking levonorgestrel*—give a replacement dose. If an anti-emetic is required, prescribe domperidone.
- *Enzyme inducing drugs,* e.g. anti-epileptics, St John's wort—efficacy may be ↓. Consider a copper-IUCD or ↑ dose of lenonorgestrel to 3 mg (1500 mcg immediately and 1500 mcg 12 h later—unlicensed).

Copper-containing IUCD: insertion of an IUCD is more effective than hormonal emergency contraception and prevents nearly 100% of pregnancies:
- Copper IUCDs (*not* Mirena®) can be inserted for emergency contraception ≤120 h (5 d) after unprotected intercourse
- Test for sexually transmitted diseases with endocervical swabs—if at risk, cover insertion with antibiotics, e.g. azithromycin 1 g stat
- If intercourse has occurred >5 d previously, the IUCD can still be inserted up to 5 d after the earliest likely calculated ovulation (i.e. within the minimum period before implantation)
- There is a small ↑ in pelvic infections in the 20 d following insertion of an IUCD.

Follow-up: 3–4 wk after prescribing emergency contraception or inserting an IUCD—sooner if heavy vaginal bleeding or pelvic pain. Include:
- Checking the patient is not pregnant—may need a pregnancy test
- Talking about regular methods of contraception that would prevent pregnancy and the need for emergency contraception in future
- Screening for sexually transmitted diseases, if needed
- If the patient is pregnant, discussing options for pregnancy.

❶ There is no evidence treatment with levonorgestrel harms the foetus.

Further information
Department of Health CMO Update 35 (2003) 🖳 www.dh.gov.uk
FFPRH Emergency contraception (2006) 🖳 www.ffprhc.org.uk

Patient advice about emergency hormonal contraception

- Contact your doctor if you vomit within 3 h of taking your emergency contraceptive pill as it will not have had time to work. Your doctor can then give you a replacement pill
- Use a barrier method of contraception until your next period
- Your next period may be early or late. You may also get some spotting before you have your next period
- If you get any lower abdominal pain or heavy bleeding or are worried in any other way, then talk to your doctor
- Go back to your doctor in 3–4 weeks if you have not had a period or your period was abnormally light, brief or heavy
- If the emergency contraceptive pill does not work, there is no evidence that it harms the baby.

If you do not use a regular contraceptive and are having unprotected intercourse, using emergency contraception is not a reliable way of preventing pregnancy. Talk to your doctor or local family planning clinic about methods of regular contraception which would be suitable for you, and ways to prevent sexually transmitted diseases.

Table 12.2 Emergency contraception for failure of contraception

Situation	Indication for emergency contraception
Combined oral contraceptive (21 active pills)	If ≥3 30–35-mcgm ethinyl oestradiol or ≥2 20-mcgm ethinylestradiol pills have been missed, vomiting/severe diarrhoea or broad-spectrum antibiotic in the first week of pill-taking (i.e. days 1–7) and unprotected intercourse in the pill-free week or week 1.
Progestogen only pills (POP)	If ≥1 POPs have been missed or taken >3 h late (>12 h late for Cerazette®) and unprotected intercourse has occurred in the 2 d following this.
Intrauterine contraception	If complete or partial expulsion is identified or midcycle removal of an IUCD/IUS has been necessary and unprotected intercourse has occurred in the last 7 d.
Progestogen only injectables	If the contraceptive injection is late (>14 wk from the previous injection for medroxyprogesterone acetate and >10 wk for norethisterone enantate) and unprotected sexual intercourse.
Barrier method	Failure of a barrier method.
Liver-enzyme inducing drugs	Patients taking the COC, POP or with a progestogen implant should use additional contraception if taking liver-enzyme inducing drugs. Use emergency contraception if barrier methods fail or there is unprotected intercourse during, or in the 28 d following, use of liver-enzyme inducing drugs.

Reproduced with permission from the Faculty of family planning and reproductive health.

☼ / ⊛ **Bleeding in pregnancy**

Bleeding up to 14 wk into pregnancy: bleeding in early pregnancy occurs in 1:4 pregnancies. *Causes:*
- Bleeding in normal pregnancy—largest group
- Miscarriage
- Ectopic pregnancy
- Trophoblastic disease
- Non-obstetric conditions, e.g. friable cervix, polyp, cervical neoplasia

⚠ Any sexually active woman presenting with abdominal pain and vaginal bleeding after an interval of amenorrhoea has an ectopic pregnancy until proven otherwise.

Assessment
- Take a history of pain and bleeding—pain preceding bleeding suggests ectopic pregnancy is more likely. Have any products of conception been passed? ❶ Clots/products can be difficult to distinguish
- Check LMP and pregnancy test result (do a test if a pregnancy test has not been done)
- Check pulse (>100 bpm suggests shocked), BP and temperature (? toxic)
- Abdominal examination—guarding, peritonism and/or unilateral tenderness suggest ectopic pregnancy
- Pelvic examination—with the advent of Early Pregnancy Assessment Units, the necessity of pelvic examination is debatable. If performed, assess uterine size, cervix—is the cervix open? (a closed cervix admits only 1 fingertip in a multiparous woman), is there any other cause for the bleeding?

Initial management
- If severe bleeding and/or pain, shocked or toxic, admit to gynaecology as an emergency. If shocked, give 1 ml syntometrine® IM and try to gain IV access.
- Otherwise, refer to the Early Pregnancy Assessment Unit (EPAU), if available, to check site and viability of pregnancy. USS is the definitive test of viability of pregnancy—at 5 wk gestation sac ± yolk sac is seen on scan; at 6 wk a foetal pole and foetal heart beat is usually seen (occasionally not seen until 7 wk). Blood group and rhesus status is also checked at the EPAU.

❶ Advise women there is a strong possibility of a transvaginal ultrasound scan (~40%)—in practice, usually well tolerated.

Bleeding in early normal pregnancy: often termed *threatened miscarriage*. If foetal heart is seen on USS then there is ~97% chance of the pregnancy continuing to progress. There is no evidence that rest or abstinence from sex improves outcome.

Complications of bleeding: significant subchorionic haematoma is associated with ↑ risk of premature rupture of membranes and IUGR—refer early for specialist antenatal care.

⚠ **Rhesus −ve women**

Bleeding <12 wk gestation: anti-D is not required for:
- Threatened miscarriage unless heavy or repeated bleeding and/or abdominal pain or
- Complete miscarriage where there is no medical or surgical uterine evacuation.

❶ If there is any clinical doubt, give anti-D.

Bleeding >12 wk gestation, ectopic pregnancy and/or medical/surgical evacuation of the uterus at any gestation: give anti-D immunoglobulin (250 iu IM if gestation <20wk) within 72 h of bleeding—whether or not the pregnancy is lost.

Dealing with psychological effects of early loss of pregnancy

- Broach the subject with all women who have suffered a miscarriage or other early loss of pregnancy—one way of doing this is to telephone the patient after discharge and offer support
- Include the woman's partner if possible
- Not all women are grieved—adjust your approach accordingly
- Legitimize any grief and acknowledge it
- Provide information about the condition which caused the loss and reassure where appropriate about the future (if <3 miscarriages, risk of further miscarriage is not significantly ↑, risk of further ectopic pregnancy is ~1:10)
- Discuss worries and concerns of the woman and her partner
- Warn of the anniversary phenomenon (sadness felt at the baby's due date or anniversary of the pregnancy loss) or sadness/jealousy they may feel on the birth of another's baby
- Inform about self-help organizations, e.g. miscarriage association, ectopic pregnancy trust
- Provide ongoing support as needed. An easy access policy is useful as different women will want to discuss their feelings at different times after loss. If the woman already has young children, inform the health visitor.

Miscarriage: also termed spontaneous abortion. Occurs in 1:5 pregnancies—80% at <12 wk gestation. *Risk factors:*
- Maternal age
- BMI >29 kg/m², —if >32 kg/m², risk is ↑ by 30%
- Smoking
- Excess alcohol

Causes
- Foetal abnormality (50%)
- Multiple pregnancy
- Uterine abnormality—fibroids, polyps, congenital abnormality, cervical incompetence (late 2nd trimester miscarriages)
- Systemic disease—renal, autoimmune or connective tissue disease—particularly SLE, PCOS, DM, systemic infection
- Drugs—cytotoxics, stilboestrol
- Placental vascular abnormalities.

Management
- *Complete miscarriage*—psychological support
- *Incomplete miscarriage*—products of conception remain in the uterus but there is no foetal heart—usually admitted for evacuation of retained products of conception (ERPC). Some women prefer a 'watch and wait' approach—at 3 d 86% will be complete.
- *Missed (or delayed) miscarriage*—usually discovered when no heart beat is seen on routine antenatal scan. Treatment is with ERPC. A 'watch and wait' approach is possible but at 4 wk, only 66% are complete, and associated with longer bleeding.

❶ Medical management with prostaglandin analogues ± antiprogesterone priming is an alternative to ERPC and offered in some units.

Rhesus-negative women: 📖 p.187.

Complications
- *Early*—Perforation of the uterus, retained products of conception, infection. Treat with antibiotics if infection is suspected (e.g. doxycycline 100 mg od). Re-refer/readmit if shock, pain, heavy bleeding or bleeding is not settling.
- *Later*—uterine synechiae (Aschermann's syndrome), cervical incompetence, psychological sequelae.

Ectopic pregnancy: a fertilized egg implants outside the uterine cavity—95% in a Fallopian tube. Incidence ≈1:100 pregnancies and increasing due to ↑ *Chlamydia* infections and PID. Risk factors—Box 12.1.

History
- *Abdominal pain (97%):* unilateral or bilateral, often starts before bleeding, may radiate to shoulder tip, ↑ on passing urine/opening bowels
- *Amenorrhoea (absent in 25%):* peak incidence after 7 wk amenorrhoea.
- *Irregular vaginal bleeding (79%):* described as 'prune juice' but may be fresh blood, usually not heavy. May pass decidual cast.

Examination
- Shock in 15–20%
- Abdominal tenderness ± rebound or guarding (71%)
- Pelvis—enlarged uterus, adnexal mass, and/or cervical excitation.

Management: admit immediately for further investigation. Resuscitate before admission as needed. Hospital management may be expectant (watch and pregnancy resolves spontaneously), medical (methotrexate) or surgical (laparotomy or laparoscopic surgery). Offer early USS in future pregnancies to confirm pregnancy is intrauterine.

Complications: death if undetected, infertility (pregnancy rate post ectopic pregnancy is 66% with 10% having a further ectopic pregnancy).

Further information

RCOG 🖳 www.rcog.org.uk
• Management of Early Pregnancy Loss (2000)
• The management of tubal pregnancy (2004)

Table 12.3 Probability of successful pregnancy after miscarriage

Age (y)	Number of previous miscarriages			
	2	3	4	5
20	92	90	88	85
25	89	86	82	79
30	84	80	76	71
35	77	73	68	62
40	69	64	58	52
45	60	54	48	42

Reproduced with permission from *The Obstetrician and Gynaecologist*, October 2000.

Box 12.1 Risk factors for ectopic pregnancy

• PID (single episode ↑ risk ×7)
• Infertility (15%)
• IUCD (14%)
• Previous ectopic pregnancy (11%)
• Tubal surgery
• POP
• Age
• Smoking

Further information/support for patients

Miscarriage Association ☎ 01924 200799 🖳 www.miscarriageassociation.org.uk
Ectopic Pregnancy Trust ☎ 01895 238025 🖳 www.ectopic.org

Antepartum haemorrhage (APH): any bleeding in pregnancy >24wk gestation (or the point of foetal viability). *Causes:*

Uterine:
- Abruption (□ p.197)
- Placenta praevia (below)
- Vasa praevia
- Circumvallate placenta
- Placental sinuses

Lower genital tract:
- Cervical
  - Polyp
  - Erosion
  - Carcinoma
  - Cervicitis
- Vaginitis
- Vulval varicosities

⚠ *Action*

- ALWAYS admit to a specialist obstetric unit. If bleeding is severe admit via an emergency ambulance and while awaiting transport raise legs; give O_2 via face mask; if possible gain IV access, take blood for FBC and cross matching and start IV infusion.
- NEVER do a vaginal examination—placenta praevia bleeds +++.

Placenta praevia: occurs when the placenta lies within the lower uterine segment. *Incidence:* 1:4 routine anomaly scans done at 19 wk gestation show a low lying placenta—5% stay low at 32 wk; <2% at term.

Associations
- ↑ with parity
- Age >35 y
- Smoking
- Twins
- Endometrial damage (e.g. history of D&C, TOP)
- Preterm delivery
- Previous LSCS
- Placental pathology (marginal/vellamentous cord insertions, succenturiate lobes, bipartite placenta)
- Previous placenta praevia (recurrence rate 4–8%).

Management: if discovered at routine USS at 17–19 wk, follow-up USS at 32 wk reveals whether the placenta is moving out of the lower segment. When the placenta remains low management depends on whether the placenta covers the internal os (major placenta praevia) or not (minor placenta praevia). Major placenta praevia always requires delivery by caesarean section. Normal delivery in a specialist unit may be attempted with minor placenta praevia if the head lies below the lower edge of the placenta.

Complications

Maternal
- APH—typically painless bleeding with a peak incidence at 34 wk
- Malpresentation—35% breech presentation or transverse lie
- Placental problems—placenta accreta and percreta especially with a history of previous caesarean section; abruption
- Postpartum haemorrhage.

Foetal: IUGR (15%); premature delivery; death.

Postpartum haemorrhage (PPH)

Primary PPH: loss of >500 ml blood within 24 h of delivery. Affects 1:100 deliveries. **Causes:** uterine atony (90%); genital tract trauma (7%); clotting disorders (3%)

Risk factors

- Past history of PPH
- Retained placenta (p.199)
- Large placental site
- Low placenta
- Overdistended uterus
- Abruption
- Uterine malformation
- Fibroids
- Prolonged labour
- >5 previous vaginal deliveries
- Trauma to uterus or cervix.

⚠ Action

- Give high flow O_2 via face mask as soon as possible.
- Call emergency ambulance for transfer to hospital.
- Gain IV access, take blood for FBC and cross matching and start IV infusion if possible.
- Give in turn as necessary oxytocin 5–10 units by slow IV injection, ergometrine 0.25–0.5 mg IV and, then if available and still bleeding, IV oxytocin infusion (5–30 units in 500 ml) given at a rate that controls uterine atony.
- If the placenta has not been delivered attempt to deliver it by controlled cord traction.
- Check for trauma and apply pressure to any visible bleeding point/repair any visible bleeding point. Bimanual pressure on the uterus may decrease immediate loss.
- Some community units keep misoprostol 400–800 mcgm and carboprost 250 mcgm in 1 ml (e.g. Haemabate) for emergency use. Give misoprostol PR and/or carboprost by deep IM injection (can be repeated after >15 min to a maximum total dose of 2 mg).

Secondary PPH: Excessive blood loss PV >24 h after delivery. *Peak incidence:* 5–12 d. after delivery. *Causes:* Retained placental tissue or clot; postpartum infection.

⚠ Action

- Refer for assessment and possible USS
- If bleeding is slight and USS normal, manage conservatively. If any suggestion of infection, take a swab and start oral antibiotics—amoxicillin 500 mg tds and metronidazole 400 mg tds until sensitivities known
- If the uterus is tender and the os open, if loss is heavy or there is any suggestion of retained products on USS, admit to an obstetric unit for further investigation/evacuation of retained products of conception.

Further information

RCOG www.rcog.org.uk
- Management of postpartum haemorrhage (1997 and update, 2002)
- Placenta previa and palcenta previa accreta: diagnosis and management (2005)

⊛ /☼ Pre-eclampsia and eclampsia

Pre-eclampsia, *Pregnancy induced hypertension and proteinuria* or *pre-eclamptic toxaemia (PET)* affects 5–7% of primigravida and 2–3% of all pregnancies. Multisystem disease of unknown cause, developing ≥20 wk into pregnancy and only resolving once the baby is delivered (<10d. after birth). *Risk factors*—Box 12.2. Untreated, may progress to eclampsia—one of the commonest causes of death from pregnancy.

Criteria for diagnosis of pre-eclampsia
- BP>140/90 or >+30/+15 from booking. The earlier in pregnancy the BP rises, the more likely the pre-eclampsia will be severe.
- Proteinuria ≥0.3 g/24 h—urine dipstick is a useful screening tool—if ≥1+ protein then probably significant—but ~25% false +ve rate.

Thresholds for further action: Table 12.4, 🕮 p.194.

⚠ *Significant symptoms/signs of pre-eclampsia*
- New hypertension
- New and/or significant proteinuria
- Maternal symptoms of headache and/or visual disturbance
- Maternal epigastric pain and/or vomiting
- Reduced foetal movements or small for gestational age infant.

Risk of recurrence
- Risk of recurrence in subsequent pregnancy with the same partner is 10–15% but usually less severe.
- Women who have pre-eclampsia are at greater risk of developing ↑BP later in life.

Eclampsia: occurs when the woman has a fit as a result of pre-eclampsia (2% women with pre-eclampsia). Incidence: 1:2000 pregnancies—44% after delivery (usually <24 h). 35% of those who have a fit will have ≥1 major complication, e.g. stroke, and 1.8% die. Usually BP is very high—but may be normal or only mildly ↑—especially if the woman is non-Caucasian. If the baby is not yet born, it becomes distressed.

Symptoms and signs of impending eclampsia
- Restlessness/agitation
- ↓ urine output
- Hyperreflexia
- Retinopathy.

⚠ *Action*
- Call for help
- Ensure the environment is safe, i.e. move any objects that could harm the woman
- Turn on to side and place in the recovery position, if possible
- Ensure airway is clear
- If available, give magnesium sulphate 4 g IV over 10–15 min then 1 g/h infusion. If not available, give one dose of diazepam 5–10 mg IV or PR
- Admit as 'blue light' emergency

Box 12.2 Risk factors for pre-eclampsia

- Pre-eclampsia/eclampsia in previous pregnancy
- Multiple pregnancy
- Underlying medical conditions:
  - Pre-existing hypertension or booking diastolic BP ≥90 mmHg
  - Pre-existing renal disease or booking proteinuria ≥1+ on >1 occasion or quantified as ≥0.3 g/24 h
  - Pre-existing DM
  - Antiphospholipid antibodies
- First pregnancy (or first time by a new partner)
- Age ≥40 y
- BMI ≥35 or <18 kg/m^2
- Family history of eclampsia/pre-eclampsia (particularly mother/sister)
- Booking diastolic BP ≥80 but <90 mmHg.

⚠ Pre-eclampsia is asymptomatic until its terminal phase, and onset may be rapid, so frequent BP screening is essential. Whenever you check BP in pregnancy, always check urine for protein.

HELLP syndrome: occurs in pregnancy or <48 h after delivery. Associated with severe pre-eclampsia.
- Haemolysis
- Elevated liver enzymes
- Low platelets.

Signs
- Hypertension (80%)
- Right upper quadrant pain (90%)
- Nausea and vomiting (50%)
- Oedema

Management: admit as for pre-eclampsia.

Table 12.4 Thresholds for further action

Findings (BP readings are in mmHg)		Action
New hypertension without proteinuria >20 wk gestation	Diastolic BP ≥90 and <100 mmHg	Refer for specialist assessment* in <48 h
	Diastolic BP ≥90 and <100 mmHg with significant symptoms (below)	Refer for same day specialist assessment*
	Diastolic BP ≥100 mmHg	
	Systolic BP ≥160 mmHg	
New hypertension and proteinuria >20 wk gestation	Diastolic BP ≥90 and new proteinuria ≥1+ on dipstick	Refer for same day specialist assessment*
	Diastolic BP ≥90 and new proteinuria ≥1+ on dipstick and significant symptoms (below)	
	Diastolic BP ≥110 and new proteinuria ≥1+ on dipstick	Immediate admission
	Systolic BP ≥170 and new proteinuria ≥1+ on dipstick	
New proteinuria without hypertension >20 wk gestation	1+ on dipstick	Repeat pre-eclampsia assessment in <1 wk
	2+ on dipstick	Refer for specialist assessment* in <48 h
	≥1+ on dipstick with significant symptoms (below)	Refer for same day specialist assessment*
Maternal symptoms or foetal signs/symptoms without new hypertension or proteinuria	Headache and/or visual disturbance with diastolic BP <90 and trace or no proteinuria	Investigate cause of headache. ↓ interval to next pre-eclampsia assessment
	Epigastric pain with diastolic BP <90 and trace or no proteinuria	If simple antacids are ineffective, refer for same day specialist assessment*
	↓ foetal movements or small for gestational age infant with diastolic BP <90 and trace or no proteinuria	Refer for investigation of foetal compromise. ↓ interval to next pre-eclampsia assessment

*Most obstetric departments have a day case 'step-up' assessment unit.

⚠ Significant symptoms:
- Epigastric pain
- Vomiting
- Headache
- Visual disturbance
- ↓ foetal movements
- Small for gestational age infant

Further information

APEC Pre-eclampsia community guideline (2004) ▣ www.apec.org.uk
RCOG Pre-eclampsia—study group recommendations (2003) ▣ www.rcog.org.uk

Table 12.4 is reproduced with permission from APEC.

Frequently asked questions about pre-eclampsia

What is eclampsia and pre-eclampsia? Pre-eclampsia usually only occurs after the 20th week of pregnancy. It causes high blood pressure and protein to leak into the urine. Eclampsia may follow on from pre-eclampsia (1 in 2000 women with pre-eclampsia). It is a type of fit (or seizure) which is a life-threatening complication of pregnancy.

Why have I got pre-eclampsia? Any pregnant woman can develop pre-eclampsia (1 in 14 pregnancies). You have increased risk if you:
- Are pregnant for the first time (1 in 30 women get pre-eclampsia), or are pregnant for the first time by a new partner.
- Have had pre-eclampsia before.
- Have a family history of pre-eclampsia. Particularly if it occurred in your mother or sister.
- Had high blood pressure before the pregnancy started.
- Are diabetic, or have systemic lupus erythematosus (SLE), or chronic kidney disease.
- Are aged below 20 or above 35.
- Have a pregnancy with twins, triplets, or more.
- Are obese.

What causes pre-eclampsia? No one really knows. It is probably due to a problem with the placenta (the afterbirth).

How do you know I have pre-eclampsia? Most women do not feel ill or have any symptoms at first. Pre-eclampsia is present if:
- your blood pressure becomes high, and
- you have an abnormal amount of protein in your urine.

Severity of pre-eclampsia is usually (but not always) related to the blood pressure level. Other symptoms which suggest severe pre-eclampsia are:
- Headaches
- Blurring of vision, or other visual problems
- Abdominal (tummy) pain—usually just below the ribs
- Vomiting
- Just not feeling right.

Swelling or puffiness of your feet, face, or hands (oedema) is also a feature of pre-eclampsia but is also common in normal pregnancy.

How is pre-eclampsia treated? Regular checks may be all that you need if pre-eclampsia remains relatively mild. If pre-eclampsia becomes worse, you are likely to be admitted to hospital. Tests may be done to check on your well-being, and that of your baby. As the only way of stopping the pre-eclampsia is to deliver the baby, in some cases babies are delivered early to prevent harm to mother or baby.

Will pre-eclampsia develop in my next pregnancy? If you had pre-eclampsia in your first pregnancy, you have about a 1 in 10 chance of it recurring in future pregnancies.

Further information

Action on Pre-EClampsia (APEC) ☎ 020 8863 3271 🖳 www.apec.org.uk

☼ /☺ **Other obstetric emergencies**

Eclampsia: 📖 p.192.

Obstetric shock: causes:
- Haemorrhage—APH (📖 p.190); placental abruption (remember—bleeding may be internal and not seen per vaginum); PPH (📖 p.191)
- Ruptured uterus—see opposite page
- Inverted uterus—📖 p.199
- Amniotic fluid embolism—see below
- Broad ligament haematoma—📖 p.199
- Pulmonary embolus—📖 p.80
- Septicaemia—📖 p.49
- Anaphylaxis (usually drugs)—📖 p.44.

⚠ *Action*
- Call for help
- Arrange immediate admission to the nearest specialist obstetric unit (or A&E, if necessary)
- Gain IV access and start IV fluids, give O₂ via face mask (if available)
- Treat the cause if apparent.

Foetal distress: signifies hypoxia. *Signs:*
- Passage of meconium during labour
- Foetal tachycardia (>160 bpm at term)
- Foetal bradycardia (<100 bpm seek urgent obstetric assistance).

⚠ *Action*
- Give the mother oxygen via a face mask
- Turn the mother on her side
- Transfer immediately to a specialist obstetric unit for further assessment ± delivery.

Amniotic fluid embolism: very rare. Mortality ~80%. Presents with profound shock, cyanosis, and dyspnoea. May occur at the height of a contraction.

⚠ *If suspected:*
- Call for help
- Resuscitate—**A**irway; **B**reathing; **C**irculation
- Transfer as a 'blue light' emergency to the nearest A&E or specialist obstetric unit.

Acute abdominal pain: non-obstetric causes of abdominal pain may be forgotten or signs may be less well localized than in the non-pregnant patient. See 📖 p.100.

Appendicitis: 1/1000 pregnancies. Mortality is higher in pregnancy and perforation commoner (15–20%). Foetal mortality is 5–10% for simple appendicitis but rises to 30% when there is perforation. Due to the pregnancy, the appendix is displaced and pain is often felt in the para-umbilical region or subcostally. Admit immediately if suspected.

Cholecystitis: 1–6/10 000 pregnancies. Pregnancy encourages gallstone formation. Symptoms include RUQ pain, nausea and vomiting. Diagnosis can be confirmed on USS. Treatment is the same as outside pregnancy aiming for interval cholecystectomy after birth.

Fibroids: torsion or red degeneration. Fibroids ↑ in size in pregnancy. They may twist if pedunculated. Red degeneration occurs usually after 20 wk and may occur until the puerperium. It presents as abdominal pain ± localized tenderness ± vomiting and low-grade fever. Confirm diagnosis with USS. Treatment is with rest and analgesia. Pain resolves within 1 wk.

Ovarian tumours/torsion: 1/1000 pregnancies. Torsion or rupture of a cyst may both cause abdominal pain as may bleeding into a cyst. USS can confirm the presence of a cyst. Management depends on the nature of the cyst and the severity of the pain. Admit for assessment.

If <20 wk gestation in addition consider:

- *Miscarriage:* 📖 p.188
- *Ectopic pregnancy:* 📖 p.188

If >20 wk in addition consider

- *Labour*
- *Abruptio placentae:* see opposite
- *Pubic symphysis dehiscence*
- *Uterine rupture:* see below
- *Haematoma of the rectus abdominis:* rarely bleeding into the rectus sheath and haematoma formation occurs spontaneously or after coughing in late pregnancy. May cause swelling and abdominal tenderness. USS can be helpful. If unsure of diagnosis admit to exclude acute surgical or obstetric cause of pain.

Abruptio placentae: 1:80–1:200 pregnancies. Part of the placenta becomes detached from the uterus. Consequences depend on the degree of separation and the amount of blood loss.

Presentation

- Typically constant pain—may be felt in the back if posterior placenta
- Woody hard, tender uterus
- Shock ± PV bleeding
- Foetal heart absent or signs of foetal distress—foetal tachycardia or bradycardia

⚠ *Action:* if suspected admit as an acute emergency to the nearest specialist obstetric unit.

Uterine rupture: rare in the UK (1:1500 deliveries). Associated with maternal mortality of 5% and foetal mortality of 30%. 70% are due to dehiscence of caesarean section scars. Rupture occurs most commonly during labour but occasionally may occur in the 3rd trimester or after an otherwise normal delivery.

Presentation: pain is variable but usually severe, bursting, constant lower abdominal pain ± heavy vaginal bleeding. Generally associated with profound shock in the mother and foetal distress. If in labour, the presenting part may disappear from the pelvis ± contractions stop.

⚠ *Action:* admit as an acute emergency to a specialist obstetric unit.

Cord prolapse: 1:200–300 births. The cord passes through the os in front of the presenting part of the baby. If the presenting part squashes the cord, umbilical blood flow is restricted causing foetal hypoxia and distress (foetal mortality 10–17%). *Risk factors:*

- Malpresentation—breech/
  transverse/oblique
- Cephalo-pelvic disproportion
- Multiple pregnancy
- Preterm rupture of membranes
- Polyhydramnios
- Pelvic tumours

⚠ **Action**
- Minimize handling of the cord to prevent spasm
- Try to keep the cord within the vagina
- Call for help
- Aim to prevent presenting part from occluding the cord. Try:
- Displacing the presenting part upwards with the examining hand
- Get patient into knee/elbow position—head down
- If possible, drop the head end of the bed
- Fill the bladder with 500–750 ml normal saline via a catheter and clamp the catheter.
- Admit as an emergency to the nearest specialist obstetric unit—usually treated with emergency Caesarean section.

Shoulder dystocia: affects <1% deliveries but is a life-threatening emergency. Occurs when the anterior shoulder impacts upon the symphysis pubis after the head has delivered and prevents the rest of the baby following. Most cases of shoulder dystocia are unanticipated.

Clues
- Prolonged 1st or 2nd stage of labour
- 'Head bobbing'—the head consistently descends then returns to its original position during a contraction or pushing in the 2nd stage.

If shoulder dystocia occurs in the community there is usually not time to transfer a woman to a specialist unit.

⚠ **Action:** call for help. Consider episiotomy. Then try any of these procedures (no particular order):
- Roll the mother on to hands and knees and try delivering posterior shoulder first.
- Flex and abduct the mother's legs up to her abdomen (upside down squatting position)—try delivery again.
- Deliver the posterior arm—put a hand in the vagina in front of the baby—ensure the posterior elbow is flexed in front of the body and pull to deliver the forearm. The anterior shoulder usually follows.
- External pressure—ask an assistant to apply suprapubic pressure with the heel of the hand—a rocking movement can help.
- Adduction of the most accessible (preferably anterior) shoulder. Simultaneously put pressure on the posterior clavicle to turn the baby. If unsuccessful continue rotation through 180° and try again.

Uterine inversion: rare.

> ⚠ *Action:* do not remove the placenta if attached until the uterus is replaced. If noted early, try to replace the uterus. Otherwise admit as an emergency. The mother may become profoundly shocked so set up an IV infusion before transfer if possible, and give O_2 via a face mask.

Retained placenta: the 3rd stage of labour is complete in <10 min in 97% of labours. If the placenta has not been delivered in <30 min (to allow for cervical spasm), it will probably not deliver spontaneously.

> ⚠ *Action*
> - Avoid excessive cord traction.
> - Check the placenta is not in the vagina—remove if it is
> - Check the uterus
>
> *If the uterus is well contracted*: cervical spasm is probably trapping an otherwise separated placenta—wait for cervix to relax to enable removal of the placenta.
>
> *If the uterus is bulky*: the placenta may have failed to separate. Try:
> - Rubbing up a contraction
> - Putting the baby to the breast (stimulates uterine contraction)
> - Giving a further dose of syntometrine
> - If the placenta will still not deliver, admit as emergency for manual removal.

Broad ligament haematoma: presents in a recently delivered woman as obstetric shock without excessive vaginal bleeding. Examination reveals pain and tenderness on the affected side. The uterus is deviated from that side.

> ⚠ *Action:* admit as an acute emergency to the nearest specialist obstetric unit.

Resuscitation of the newborn

Resuscitation of the newborn: follow the algorithm in Figure 12.1.

Rapid assessment of the infant at birth: start the clock. Assess colour, tone, breathing, heart rate.

A healthy baby
- Born blue
- Good tone
- Cries seconds after delivery
- Good heart rate (120–150 bpm)
- Rapidly becomes pink during the first 90 sec.

A less healthy baby
- Blue at birth
- Less good tone
- ± slow heart rate (<100 bpm)
- ± inadequate breathing by 90–120 sec.

An ill baby
- Born pale
- Floppy
- Slow/very slow heart rate (<100 bpm)
- Not breathing.

Heart rate: best judged by listening with a stethoscope—in many cases it can also be felt by palpating the umbilical cord—feeling for peripheral pulses is not helpful.

Airway
- Open the airway by placing the head in a neutral position—where the neck is neither extended nor flexed.
- If the occiput is prominent and the neck tends to flex, place a support under the shoulders—but don't overextend the neck.
- If the baby is very floppy, apply jaw thrust or chin lift as needed.

Breathing: inflation breaths are breaths with pressures of ~30 cm of water for 2–3 sec.

If heart rate ↑: you have successfully inflated the chest. If the baby doesn't then start breathing alone, continue to provide regular breaths at a rate of ~30–40 breaths/min until the baby starts to breathe on its own.

If heart rate does not ↑: either you have not inflated the chest or the baby needs more help. By far the most likely is that you have failed to inflate the chest (the chest does not move). *Consider:*
- Is the baby's head in the neutral position?
- Do you need jaw thrust?
- Do you need a longer inflation time?
- Do you need a second person's help with the airway?
- Is there an obstruction in the oropharynx, e.g. meconium (laryngo-scope and suction)?
- What about an oropharyngeal (Guedel) airway?

Chest compressions: only commence after inflation of the lungs.
- Grip the chest in both hands in such a way that the thumbs of both hands can press on the sternum at a point just below an imaginary line joining the nipples and with the fingers over the spine at the back.
- Compress the chest quickly—↓ the AP diameter of the chest by ~$^1/_3$ with each compression. The ratio of compressions to inflations is 3:1.

Drug support: for a few babies inflation of the lungs and effective chest compression is not sufficient to produce effective circulation. IV or interosseous drugs may be helpful. *Doses:*
- Adrenaline: 10 mcgm/kg (0.1 ml/kg of 1:10 000 solution) increasing to 30 mcgm/kg (0.3 ml/kg of 1:10 000 solution) if ineffective
- Sodium bicarbonate: 1–2 mmol/kg (2–4 ml 4.2% bicarbonate solution)
- Dextrose: 250 mg/kg (2.5 ml/kg of 10% dextrose)

For emergency volume replacement (e.g. history of a bleed)—use 10 ml/kg 0.9% saline given over 10–20 sec. Repeat if needed.

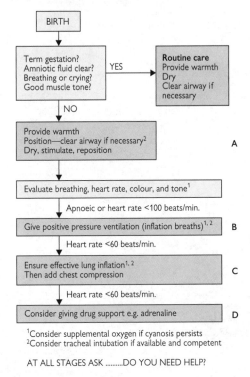

^{1}Consider supplemental oxygen if cyanosis persists
^{2}Consider tracheal intubation if available and competent

AT ALL STAGES ASK ....DO YOU NEED HELP?

Fig. 12.1 Newborn life support algorithm.

Further information

Resuscitation Council (UK) Resuscitation guidelines (2005) 🖳 www.resus.org.uk

Injuries and accidents

◉ **Neck problems**

⚠ **Neck trauma:** any significant cervical trauma requires neck immobilization with a hard collar and referral to A&E for cervical spine X-rays to exclude vertebral fracture or instability that could threaten the spinal cord.

Neck pain is common (lifetime incidence 50%) and contributes to 2% of GP consultations. Prevalence is highest in middle age. Most neck pain is acute and self-limiting (within days/weeks) but 1:3 patients presenting to the GP with neck pain have symptoms lasting >6 mo or recurring pain.

History
- Pain—onset, site, radiation, aggravating and relieving factors, timing.
- Stiffness—timing—continuous? worse in the mornings?
- Deformity—e.g. torticollis. Onset, changes.
- Neurological symptoms—numbness, paraesthesiae, weakness.
- Other symptoms—weight loss, bowel/bladder dysfunction, sweats.

❶ Pain is often poorly localized and neck problems commonly present with shoulder pain and/or headache (cervicogenic headache) so diagnosis may be difficult.

Examination
- *Look*
  - Posture
  - Deformity, e.g. torticollis, asymmetry of scapulae.
  - Arms and hands—wasting, fasciculation? Leg weakness?
- *Feel*
  - Tenderness? Midline tenderness may be due to supraspinous or spinous process damage following a whiplash injury. Paraspinal tenderness ± spasm radiating into the trapezius is common with cervical spondylosis.
  - Crepitation—common with cervical spondylosis
- *Move/measure:* normal ranges:
  - Flexion/extension—130° total range
  - Lateral flexion—45° in each direction from a neutral position.
  - Rotation—80° in each direction from a neutral position
- *Neurology:* weakness in the upper limbs in a segmental distribution, with loss of dermatomal sensation and altered reflexes indicates a root lesion (Table 13.1). If cervical cord compression is suspected, examine the lower limbs looking for upgoing planters and hyperreflexia.

Cervical spondylosis
- Degenerative disease of the cervical spine can cause pain but minor changes are normal (especially >40 y) and usually asymptomatic.
- Pain is usually intermittent and related to activity.
- Examination reveals ↓ neck mobility. Severe degeneration can cause nerve root signs.
- Treat with analgesia ± cervical collar.

X-ray only if conservative measures fail, troublesome pain, nerve root signs or the patient has psoriasis (?psoriatic arthropathy).

Table 13.1 Neurology associated with cervical nerve root entrapment

Root	Sensory changes	Motor weakness	Reflex changes
C5	Lateral arm	Shoulder abduction/ flexion	Biceps
		Elbow flexion	
C6	Lateral forearm	Elbow flexion	Biceps
	Thumb	Wrist extension	Supinator
	Index finger		
C7	Middle finger	Elbow extension	Triceps
		Wrist flexion	
		Finger extension	
C8	Medial side of lower forearm	Finger flexion	None
	Ring and little fingers		
T1	Medial side of upper forearm	Finger abduction/ adduction	None

---

Don't forget other causes of neck pain, e.g.

- Shoulder problems
- Temporomandibular joint problems
- Ankylosing spondylitis and psoriatic spondylitis
- Rheumatoid arthritis
- Polymyalgia rheumatica
- Calcium pyrophosphate dihydrate disease (pseudogout)
- Diffuse idiopathic skeletal hyperostosis (DISH)
- Fibromyalgia
- Myeloma
- Metastatic disease
- Infection—e.g. staphylococcal, TB
- Osteomalacia.

Nerve root irritation or entrapment: secondary to degeneration, vertebral displacement or collapse, disc prolapse, local tumour or abscess. Causes neck stiffness, pain in arms or fingers, ↓ reflexes, sensory loss and ↓ power. The level of entrapment can usually be determined clinically (📖 p.205). In order of frequency:

- $C_{5/6}$—affects thumb sensation and biceps muscle power
- $C_{7/8}/T_1$—affects little finger sensation and flexor carpi ulnaris power
- $C_{6/7}$—affects middle finger sensation, triceps reflex may be absent and latissimus dorsi weak.
- $C_{4/5}$—gives shoulder pain and upper arm weakness

Management
- Analgesia ± cervical collar.
- X-ray cervical spine—lateral or oblique views.
- Refer for physiotherapy.
- Refer for further investigations (e.g. MRI) if conservative management fails and there is objective evidence of a root lesion.

⚠ Refer urgently if there are signs of spinal cord compression:
- Root pain and lower motor neurone signs at the level of the lesion *and*
- Spastic weakness, brisk reflexes, upgoing plantars, loss of co-ordination and sensation below the lesion.

Spasmodic torticollis (wry neck): common. Sudden onset painful stiff neck due to spasm of trapezius and sternocleidomastoid muscles. Self-limiting. Heat, gentle mobilization, muscle relaxants and analgesia can speed recovery. A cervical collar may help in the short-term but can prolong symptoms. Often caused by poor posture—e.g. computer-seating position; carrying heavy uneven loads.

Cervical rib: congenital condition—C7 vertebra costal process enlargement. Usually asymptomatic but can cause thoracic outlet compression leading to hand or forearm pain, weakness or numbness and thenar or hypothenar wasting. Radial pulse may be weak.

Management: X-ray of thoracic outlet may show cervical rib—but symptoms are sometimes due to fibrous bands that are not seen on X-ray. Refer to upper limb orthopaedic surgeon for further assessment.

Whiplash injuries: neck pain due to stretching or tearing of cervical muscles and ligaments due to sudden extension of neck—often due to a RTA. Pain and ↓ neck mobility typically starts several hours or days after injury. Pain may radiate to shoulders, arms and head.

Management
- Examine carefully to exclude bony tenderness requiring X-ray.
- Treat with analgesia and early mobilization—collar may help initially but avoid long-term use.
- Recovery is often slow and 40% patients suffer long-lasting symptoms. As a general rule of thumb, the quicker the symptoms develop, the longer they will take to disappear.
- Early physiotherapy, if available, can improve recovery rate
- Psychological problems and medico-legal issues can affect progress.

Self-help for neck pain and whiplash

In the first 24 h: an ice pack applied to the neck will help to relieve inflammation. Bags of frozen peas make particularly good ice packs because they mould to the body.

- First wrap the ice pack in a towel or cloth to avoid direct contact between the skin and the ice.
- Lie in bed with your head resting on a pillow and the ice pack between the pillow and your neck for 20 min at a time.

Painkillers: try normal painkillers you can buy from the chemist such as paracetamol or ibuprofen. Taken them regularly for the first few days and then as needed. If these don't help, consult your GP.

Exercise: research shows that people recover more quickly from whiplash and neck pain if they keep mobile. Here are some exercises you could try.

- Stand against a door or a wall with your head facing forward and move your eyes so you look towards the 2, 4, 8 and 10 o'clock positions. Repeat this a few times.
- Beach ball/soft ball exercises: place a ball between the wall and your forehead and then try to move it around on the wall in circles or figures of eights. Repeat the exercise, this time placing the ball between the back of your head and the wall.
- Next, take a step forward and perform the following movements.
  - Keep your face straight and upright. Draw your head back and the chin down slightly—rather like a sergeant major.
  - Draw your chin in towards your neck and bend your head carefully forward until you are looking at the floor. Return to the starting position. Repeat slowly 5 times.
  - Bend your head backwards far enough to look at the ceiling. Return to the starting position.
  - Tilt your head sideways, so the right ear is near the right shoulder. If possible try to keep your eyes looking at a fixed point straight ahead. Return to the starting position.
  - Repeat this action with the head tilted to the other side.
  - Turn your head as if trying to look backwards over your shoulder, first to the left 5 times, and then to the right 5 times. Imagine following a horizontal line on the wall at eye level.
- Lastly, loosen up your shoulders. Shrug as far up as you easily can and then downwards further than normal. Bring your shoulders to the front as if you are trying to get them to meet at the middle then brace them right back, pulling your shoulder blades together. Repeat this manoeuvre 5 times slowly.

⚠ If any of exercise makes the pain worse or cause dizziness—stop that exercise. If symptoms are not improving within 2 weeks, go to see your doctor to discuss if a physiotherapy referral would be worthwhile.

◉ Low back pain

- *Acute low back pain:* new episode of low back pain of <6 wk duration. Common—lifetime prevalence 58%
- *Chronic low back pain:* back pain lasting >3mo. If present >1y. → poor prognosis.

Causes of back pain: Table 13.2.

History: Ask:
- Circumstances of pain—history of injury; duration
- Nature and severity of pain—pain/stiffness mainly at rest or at night, easing with movement suggests inflammation, e.g. discitis, spondyloarthropathy
- Associated symptoms, e.g. numbness, weakness, bowel or bladder symptoms
- PMH—past illnesses (e.g. carcinoma), previous back problems.
- Exclude pain not coming from the back. (e.g. GI or GU pain).

Examination
- Look for deformity, e.g. kyphosis (typical of ankylosing spondylitis), loss of lumbar lordosis (common in acute mechanical back pain), scoliosis.
- Palpate lumbar vertebrae for tenderness or step deformity. Palpate for muscle spasm.
- Assess flexion, extension, lateral flexion, and rotation of the back while standing.
- Ask to lie down—this gives a good indication of severity of symptoms.
- In lower limbs look for muscle wasting and check power, sensory loss and reflexes (knee jerk and ankle jerk). Assess straight leg raise (SLR)—sciatica is present if SLR on one side elicits back/buttock pain (usually ipsilateral but can be either side) compared with SLR on the other side.

⚠ **'Red flags'**
- <20 or >55 y
- Non-mechanical pain
- Pain that worsens when supine
- Night-time pain
- Thoracic pain
- Past history of carcinoma
- HIV
- Immune suppression
- IV drug use
- Taking steroids
- Unwell
- Weight ↓
- Widespread neurology
- Structural deformity

Management of acute pain in the community: triage according to history and examination—Figure 13.1, 📖 p.211.

❶ *Do not X-ray routinely:* X-rays require a high radiation dose and +ve findings are rare. *Exceptions:*
- No improvement in >6 wk.
- Young (<25 y)—X-ray SI joints to exclude ankylosing spondylitis
- Elderly—to exclude vertebral collapse/malignancy
- History of trauma
- 'Red flag' signs

Table 13.2 Causes of back pain: age suggests the most likely cause

Age (y)	Causes	
15–30	• Postural	• Fracture
	• Mechanical	• Ankylosing spondylosis
	• Prolapsed disc	• Spondylolisthesis
	• Trauma	• Pregnancy
30–50	• Postural	• Discitis
	• Degenerative joint disease	• Spondyloarthropathies
	• Prolapsed disc	
>50	• Postural	• Malignancy (lung, breast, prostate, thyroid, kidney)
	• Degenerative	• Myeloma
	• Osteoporotic collapse	
	• Paget's disease	
Other causes	• Referred pain	• Cauda equina tumours
	• Spinal stenosis	• Spinal infection

Table 13.3 Neurology associated with lumbosacral nerve root entrapment

Root	Sensory changes	Motor weakness	Reflex changes
L2	Front of thigh	Hip flexion/adduction	None
L3	Inner thigh	Knee extension	Knee
L4	Inner shin	Knee extension Foot dorsiflexion	Knee
L5	Outer shin Dorsum of foot	Knee flexion Foot inversion Big toe dorsiflexion	None
S1	Lateral side of foot/sole	Knee flexion Foot plantarflexion	Ankle

For patients who don't require immediate referral
- *Explain the likely natural history* of the pain and advise to avoid bed rest and try to maintain normal activities (↓ chance of chronic pain).
- *Prescribe analgesia*, e.g. paracetamol ± NSAIDs and suggest self-help exercises (🕮 p.212–213)
- *Consider referral for physiotherapy, chiropractic or osteopathy*—refer patients with nerve root irritation or simple backache not returning to normal activities by 6 wk for back exercises (if available locally) or physiotherapy, chiropractic or osteopathy. Refer sooner if in a lot of pain. Do not refer if there is any possible serious pathology.

Cauda equina syndrome: results from compression of the cauda equina below L2, e.g. by disc protrusion at L4/5.

Presentation
- Numbness of the buttocks and backs of thighs
- Urinary/faecal incontinence
- Lower motor neurone weakness—signs depend on level at which the cauda equine is compressed:
  - L4: loss of dorsiflexion of the foot (and toes: L4/5)
  - S1: loss of ankle reflex, plantarflexion and eversion of the foot

Management: refer/admit as a neurological emergency. Rapid surgical intervention increases the chance of full motor and sphincter recovery.

Spinal cord compression in cancer patients: affects 5% of cancer patients—70% in the thoracic region. Presentation can be subtle. Maintain a *high* level of suspicion in all cancer patients who complain of back pain—especially those with known bony metastases or tumours likely to metastasize to bone.

Presentation
- Often back pain, worse on movement, appears before neurology.
- Neurological symptoms/signs can be non-specific—constipation, weak legs, urinary hesitancy.
- Lesions above L1 (lower end of spinal cord) may produce upper motor neurone signs (e.g. ↑ tone and reflexes) and a sensory level
- Lesions below L1 may produce lower motor neurone signs (↓ tone and reflexes) and peri-anal numbness (cauda equina syndrome).

Management: prompt treatment (<24–48 h from 1st neurological symptoms) is needed if there is any hope of restoring function. Once paralysed, <5% walk again. Treat with oral dexamethasone 16 mg/d and refer urgently for assessment and surgery/radiotherapy unless in final stages of disease.

Further information

PRODIGY Guidance on lower back pain 🖳 www.cks.library.nhs.uk

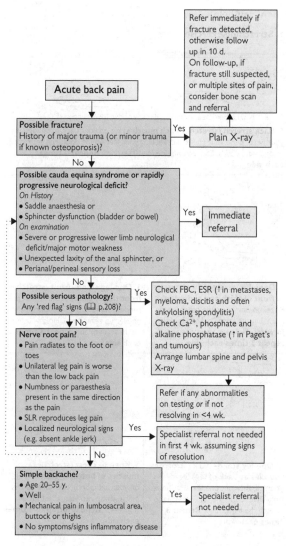

Fig. 13.1 Triage of acute back pain.

Patient self-help exercises

1. Stretching exercise

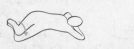

NB. Upper knee should be directly above lower knee

1. Back stretch (stretches back muscles) Lie on your back, hands above your head. Bend your knees and, keeping your feet on the floor, roll your knees to one side, slowly. Stay on one side for 10 seconds. **Repeat 3 times each side**.

2. Deep lunge (stretches muscles in front of thigh and abdomen) Kneel on one knee, the other foot in front. Lift the knee up; keep looking forwards. Hold for 5 seconds and **repeat 3 times each side**.

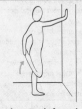

3. One-leg stand– front (stretches front thigh) Steady yourself with one hand on something for support. Bend one leg up behind you. Hold your foot for 10 seconds and **repeat 3 times each side**.

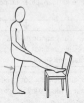

4. One-leg stand– back (stretches muscles at back of leg) Steady yourself, then put one leg, straight, up on a chair. Bend the other knee in to stretch the hamstrings. **Repeat 3 times each side**.

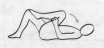

5. Knee to chest (stretches muscles of bottom– gluteals) Lie on your back. Bring one knee up and pull it gently into your chest for 5 seconds. **Repeat for up to 5 times each side**.

2. Strength, stamina and stabilizing exercises

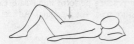

1. Pelvic tilt Lie down with your knees bent. Tighten your stomach muscles, flattening your back against the floor. Hold for 5 seconds. **Repeat 5 times**.

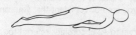

2. Stomach tone ('transverse tummy') Lie on your front with your arms by your side, head on one side. Pull in your stomach muscles, centred around your tummy button. Hold for 5 seconds. **Repeat 3 times**. Build up to 10 seconds and repeat during the day, while walking or standing. Keep breathing during this exercise.

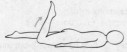

3. Buttock tone (gluteals) Bend one leg up behind you while lying on your front. Then lift your bent knee just off the floor. Hold for up to 8 seconds. **Repeat 5 times each side**.

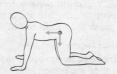

4. Deep stomach muscle tone (stabilizes lolwer back) Kneel on all fours with a small curve in your lower back. Let your stomach relax completely. Pull the lowerpart of your stomach upwards so that you lift your back (without arching it) away from the floor. Hold for 10 seconds. Keep breathing! **Repeat 10 times**.

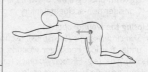

5. Back stabilizer Kneel on all fours with your back straight. Tighten your stomach. Keeping your back in position, raise one arm in front of you and hold for 10 seconds. Try to keep your pelvis level and do not rotate your body. **Repeat 10 times each side**. To progress, try lifting one leg behind you instead of your arm.

⊚ Common injuries and accidents

Wounds: most patients with significant lacerations present directly to A&E. If a patient presents to general practice perform immediate care (elevate bleeding limb and apply pressure to arrest bleeding). Advise nil by mouth and transfer to A&E.

Minor lacerations

- Ensure no foreign body is in the wound—if in doubt refer for X-ray/ surgical exploration (especially important if injury was with glass).
- Wash wound and clean away debris and any necrotic material.
- Check there is no damage to underlying nerves, tendons, bone or blood supply before dressing or closing a wound.
- Aim to oppose the skin edges without tension to allow healing.
- Do not attempt to close a wound if you are not confident that you can achieve an adequate result.
- Always refer cuts through the lip margin to A&E; consider referral to A&E for any facial wounds and wounds in children.
- Check tetanus status (Figure 13.2).
- In assault cases take particular care to document all injuries carefully, e.g. with photographs, drawings and measurements of wounds.
- Consider non-accidental injury in children—🕮 p.126.

Closing the wound: options:

- *Skin closure strips (Steristrips):* use for small cuts in non-hairy skin not under tension. For larger wounds, can be used in addition to sutures.
- *Skin 'glue' (e.g. Histoacryl):* quick (takes 30 sec to set) and can be used on hairy skin such as the scalp.
- *Suturing:* undertake training before attempting suturing.
  - Infiltrate wound edges with 1% lidocaine (max. dose—adult 200 mg; child 3 mg/kg).
  - Addition of adrenaline (epinephrine) can help haemostasis but must not be used on digits or extremities as necrosis can occur.
  - Take care to oppose edges accurately—start interrupted sutures in the middle of the wound.
  - Use appropriate suture (e.g. adult face 5-0 monofilament nylon— remove after 5 d; limbs or trunk 3-0 nylon—remove after 12 d).

Pretibial lacerations: the shin has poor blood supply especially in the elderly. Flap wounds are common, may heal poorly ± break down to form ulcers. *Management*: wash wound. Carefully realign the flap, secure with steristrips without tension and bandage. Advise elevation of the leg. Review regularly to check healing.

Nail injuries

- *Avulsed nail:* protect the nail bed of an avulsed nail with soft paraffin and gauze, check tetanus status and give antibiotic prophylaxis (e.g. flucloxacillin 250 mg qds for 5 d). Partially avulsed nails need removing under ring block to exclude an underlying nail bed injury—replace the avulsed nail in its usual position to act as a splint to the nail matrix.

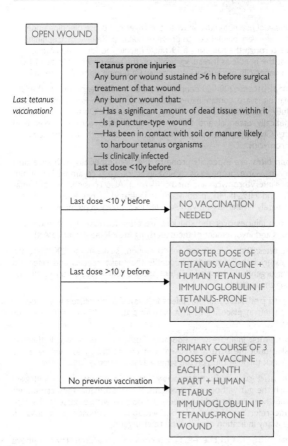

OPEN WOUND

Last tetanus vaccination?

Tetanus prone injuries
Any burn or wound sustained >6 h before surgical treatment of that wound
Any burn or wound that:
—Has a significant amount of dead tissue within it
—Is a puncture-type wound
—Has been in contact with soil or manure likely to harbour tetanus organisms
—Is clinically infected
Last dose <10y before

Last dose <10 y before → NO VACCINATION NEEDED

Last dose >10 y before → BOOSTER DOSE OF TETANUS VACCINE + HUMAN TETANUS IMMUNOGLOBULIN IF TETANUS-PRONE WOUND

No previous vaccination → PRIMARY COURSE OF 3 DOSES OF VACCINE EACH 1 MONTH APART + HUMAN TETABUS IMMUNOGLOBULIN IF TETANUS-PRONE WOUND

Fig. 13.2 Who should have tetanus vaccination?

- *Subungual haematoma:* a blow to the finger can cause bleeding under the nail—very painful due to pressure build up. Relieve by trephining a hole through the nail using a 19-gauge needle (no force required just twist the needle as it rests vertically on the nail) or a heated point (e.g. of a paper clip or cautery instrument). Of benefit up to 2 d after injury.

Animal bites: ~200 000 people are bitten by dogs each year in the UK. Animal bites are contaminated and wound infection is common. Clean carefully with soap and water. Check tetanus status. Do not suture unless cosmetically essential and there is minimal tissue damage—refer if in doubt. Give prophylaxis against infection (e.g. with co-amoxiclav or erythromycin).

Human bites: are especially prone to infection, especially with anaerobic organisms. Give prophylaxis against infection (e.g. co-amoxiclav or flu-cloxacillin/erythromycin and metronidazole). Also consider risk of Hepatitis B and HIV. If HIV prophylaxis is indicated, it needs to be started immediately—refer urgently to A&E for local policy implementation.

❶ Punch injuries over the knuckles are often associated with tooth lacerations and involvement of the underlying MCP joint—refer to A&E.

Snake bites: the adder is the only poisonous snake in the UK. Bites are only rarely lethal. Attempt to identify the snake species and refer the patient urgently to hospital. Do not apply a tourniquet or try cutting or sucking the wound.

Air gun pellets: common. Refer for X-ray. Can be difficult to remove—may be left in place if not in a harmful position. If in a joint, refer for removal.

Fish hooks: infiltrate with lidocaine. Push the hook forwards through the skin until the barb is exposed. Cut the barb off and then ease the hook back through the skin the same way it entered.

Coin and other foreign body ingestion: most coins will pass through the gut without any problems. If asymptomatic, they can be left to take their course (advise checking stools to ensure passed). If symptomatic refer for X-ray and consideration for endoscopic removal. If there is any indication of aspiration refer urgently.

Foreign bodies in the ear: most common in children. Try to remove under direct vision with forceps but avoid pushing objects deeper into the canal and causing damage. Don't poke around with forceps in an uncooperative child. Removal under GA may be needed. Insects can be drowned in oil and syringed out.

Foreign bodies in the nose: common in young children. Refer all children with unilateral offensive discharge for exploration under GA. Do not try to remove a foreign body yourself unless the object is very superficial and the child co-operative. You might push the object further in and cause trauma.

Removal of ticks: use a commercially available tick remover or place a large blob of petroleum jelly (Vaseline™) over the tick. It suffocates over a few hours and can be removed easily with a pair of tweezers.

Weaver fish sting: common on sandy beaches. The fish lurks under the sand so usually trodden on—presents with severe pain in the foot. Immerse the affected area in uncomfortably hot (but not scalding) water. Give analgesia. Pain resolves after 2–3 d.

Insect stings and bites: response depends on the insect involved and the individual's response to the stings. Ranges from blisters through papules to urticarial weals—2° infection is common.

Management

Anaphylaxis: follow algorithm in Figures 3.5 and 3.6, 📖 p.46–47, and admit to hospital as a blue light emergency.

Immediately after the sting: remove any sting present in the wound; often no further treatment is needed.
- *If severe local reaction occurs*—apply an ice pack; give oral antihistamine (e.g. chlorphenamine 4 mg stat); continue antihistamine 4–6 hourly as needed.
- *If 2° bacterial infection occurs*—treat with oral or topical antibiotics.

Remove sources of insects, e.g. remove fleas from carpets with household flea spray (multiple bites on ankles and lower legs).

Jelly fish sting
- Remove the patient from the sea as soon as possible.
- Scrape or wash adherent tentacles off.
- Alcoholic solutions including suntan lotions should **not** be applied because they may cause further discharge of stinging hairs.
- Ice packs ↓ pain and a slurry of baking soda (sodium bicarbonate), but not vinegar, may be useful for treating stings from UK species

---

Removing a tight ring from a swollen finger
- Wind cotton tape around the finger advancing towards the ring.
- Then thread tape through the ring and pull on this end to unwind the tape (levers ring over PIP joint).
- If unsuccessful, use a ring cutter

Muscle injuries and sprains: take a history and examine the patient to confirm the diagnosis and exclude fracture or dislocation.

Management
- *Rest:* relative rest of the affected part while continuing other activities to maintain overall fitness.
- *Ice and analgesia:* use immediately after injury (wrap ice in a towel and use for maximum 10 min at a time to prevent acute cold injury). Suitable analgesia is paracetamol 1 g qds and/or ibuprofen 400 mg tds/qds.
- *Compression:* taping or strapping can be used to treat (↓ swelling) and also to prevent acute sprains and strains.
- *Elevation:* ↓ local swelling and dependent oedema enabling quicker recovery.

Follow-up: if not settling in 6 wk, refer to physiotherapy (sooner if athlete, or injury preventing work).

Muscle injuries
- *Haematoma* within or between muscles can → dramatic whole limb bruising (due to tracking of blood) and stiffness. Treat with RICE regime (see above), encourage movement in pain-free range.
- *Strain* (e.g. hamstring injury). Refer to physiotherapy. A secondary injury is likely if the patient returns to sport too soon.

Ligament injuries (sprains)
- *Grade 1*—local tenderness, normal joint movement. Give NSAIDs, support strain, encourage mobilization.
- *Grade 2*—slightly abnormal joint movement. More joint protection, NSAIDs, elevate limb, encourage middle of the range movement,
- *Grade 3*—abnormal joint movement. Refer to orthopaedics.

Shoulder dislocation: usually due to fall on arm or shoulder—anterior dislocation is most common.
- Shoulder contour is lost (flattening of deltoid) and the head of the humerus is seen as an anterior bulge.
- Axillary nerve may be damaged → absent sensation on a patch below the shoulder.
- Occasionally immediate reduction is possible (i.e. on the sports field) but beware of concurrent fractures—refer to A&E for X-ray and reduction.
- In young patients, ~ 30% have recurrent dislocations afterwards due to labral tear.
- Dislocation is associated with rotator cuff tear in ~25% of elderly patients.

Recurrent dislocation: usually anterior and follows trauma—but 5% recurrent dislocations are in teenagers with no history of trauma but general joint laxity. Refer for specialist physiotherapy and consideration of surgery.

Dislocation of the jaw: 📖 p.227.

Mallet finger: the fingertip droops due to avulsion of the extensor tendon attachment to the terminal phalanx (Figure 13.3). Refer for X-ray.

Management: a plastic splint which holds the terminal phalanx in extension is worn for 6 wk to help union (must not be removed). Arthrodesis may be needed if healing doesn't occur.

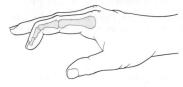

Fig. 13.3 Mallet finger.

Gamekeeper thumb: forced thumb abduction causes rupture of the ulnar collateral ligament. Can occur on wringing pheasants' necks (chronic slow stretch of ligament)—hence the name, or, more commonly, acutely by catching the thumb in the matting on a dry ski slope. The thumb is very painful and pincer grip weak. Refer—open surgical repair is the most effective treatment.

Fractures
- *Symptoms:* pain at the affected site—worse on movement, ↓ function.
- *Signs:* swelling; bruising; deformity; local tenderness; impaired function; crepitus; abnormal mobility.

⚠ **Action**
- Immobilize the affected part and give analgesia
- If available and the patient is shocked, start an IV infusion
- Refer to A&E for assessment, X-ray and treatment.

Head and facial injury: 🕮 p.222.
Ankle or foot injury: Box 13.1, 🕮 p.220.
Common fractures seen in primary care: Table 13.4, 🕮 p.221.

⚠ Always consider assessment and treatment for osteoporosis in all men and women >50 y who have had a Colles' fracture, hip fracture and/or vertebral collapse.

Fracture complications: often occur after the patient has been discharged from hospital and may present as a primary care emergency. Patients should not have persistent pain—beware of compartment syndrome (🕮 p.220). Refer back to the fracture clinic or A&E if:
- Persistent pain
- Limb swelling that is not settling
- Offensive odour or discharge
- If cast edges are abrading the skin or if the cast has deteriorated in structural strength, e.g. from getting wet

Compartment syndrome: crush injury, fracture, prolonged immobility or tight splints, dressings or casts can result in ↑ pressure within muscle compartments and ultimately → vascular occlusion. Hypoxia and necrosis cause further ↑ pressure.

Signs: swelling, severe pain—↑ on passive stretch of muscles, distal numbness, redness, mottling, blisters. ❶ pulses may be present distally.

Action: loosen any restricting bandage or cast. Refer as an emergency for orthopaedic assessment—a fasciotomy may be needed to relieve the pressure.

Box 13.1 Ottawa rules for ankle or foot injury

Twisting of the ankle resulting in pain and swelling is a very common injury. Foot injuries are also common. It can be difficult to distinguish between a sprain and a fracture. The Ottawa rules ↓ need for X-ray by ¼:

Ankle injury: refer for an ankle X-ray if there is pain in the malleolar area AND
- bone tenderness at the posterior tip of the lateral malleolus, or
- bone tenderness at the posterior tip of the medial malleolus, or
- patient is unable to weight bear at the time of the injury and when seen.

Foot injury: refer for a foot X-ray if there is pain in the midfoot AND
- bone tenderness at the 5th metatarsal base, or
- bone tenderness at the navicular, or
- patient is unable to weight bear at the time of injury and when seen.

Otherwise diagnose a sprain: treat sprains with rest, ice, compression, elevation and analgesia (paracetamol ± NSAIDs). If severe (or the patient is an athlete), refer to physiotherapy.

Table 13.4 Common fractures seen in primary care

Fracture	Features and management
Clavicle	Common injury (5% all fractures). Usually results from a fall on to an outstretched arm. 80% fractures are in the middle $^1/_3$; 15% the lateral $^1/_3$ and 5% the medial $^1/_3$.
	Refer to A&E for confirmation of diagnosis and fracture clinic follow-up. Treatment is with sling support and analgesia. Most heal well.
	Complications: pneumothorax, malunion, and nerve/vessel damage.
Colles'	Most commonly due to a fall on to an outstretched hand in an elderly lady. Pain and swelling of the wrist ('dinner-fork' deformity).
	Refer any suspected fracture for X-ray and reduction.
	Complications: include rupture of the extensor pollicis longus tendon, carpal tunnel syndrome and reflex sympathetic dystrophy
Scaphoid	Caused by falling onto an outstretched hand. Pain, swelling and tenderness in the anatomical snuff box.
	Symptoms may be mild and fracture is easily missed—refer suspected cases for scaphoid view X-rays. If X-ray is inconclusive and pain continues, repeat 2 wk later—bone scan or MRI can help if still –ve.
	Non-union and avascular necrosis of the proximal fragment is a potential complication, which can lead to long-term problems of arthritis and pain.
Fingers	Common injuries. Often associated with sport. Refer all suspected fractures for X-ray ± reduction
Hip	Common among the elderly and carries high morbidity and mortality (≈25%). ♀ > ♂. Usually occurs through the neck of the femur.
	Risk factors: maternal hip fracture, osteoporosis, unsteadiness, sedative medication, poor eye sight and polypharmacy.
	There may be a history of a fall but not always. Suspect in any patient who is elderly or has risk factors for osteoporosis who is 'off legs'. Occasionally patients can still weight bear with difficulty.
	Signs: External rotation, shortening and adduction of leg.
	Refer urgently to A&E for X-ray.
Ankle	History is of a fall over an obstacle or trip down a step. The ankle rapidly becomes swollen and tender—often on both sides.
	Decide whether an X-ray is needed (Box 13.1). If so, refer to A&E.
Metatarsals	The most common fracture is of the base of the 5th metatarsal in an 'ankle twisting' injury. March or stress fractures occur in people who do a lot of walking or running and affect the neck/shaft of the 2nd metatarsal.
	Decide whether an X-ray is needed (Box 13.1). If so, refer to A&E. Undisplaced fractures are usually treated with analgesia and support.
Toes	Caused by stubbing the toe or dropping a heavy object on it.
	Undisplaced suspected fractures: Do not X-ray unless diagnosis is in doubt. Support the injured toe by 'buddy' strapping it to the adjacent toe. Give analgesia.
	Fracture displacement and/or dislocation: Refer for X-ray and reduction.

☺ **Head injury**

Severe head injury
- Perform basic life support (📖 p.18)
- Protect the cervical spine (see below and 📖 p.204)
- Transfer to A&E by ambulance.

Less severe head injuries

History: if possible take the history from a witness as well as the patient. Ask about circumstances of injury, loss of consciousness (LOC), seizures, current symptoms and behaviour.

Examination: check scalp, head for injury, neurological examination (including fundi), other injuries—accompanying neck injuries are common.

⚠ *Refer to A&E if:*
- Glasgow Coma Scale <15 at any time since injury (Table 13.5)
- Loss of consciousness
- Focal neurological deficit since injury—problems speaking, understanding, reading, writing, ↓ sensation, loss of balance, weakness, visual changes, abnormal reflexes, problems walking, irritability or altered behaviour especially in young children
- Any suspicion of skull fracture; penetrating head injury; blood or CSF in the nose, ear or wound; serious scalp laceration or haematoma
- Amnesia for events before or after injury
- Persistent headache
- Vomiting
- Seizure
- Any previous cranial neurosurgical interventions
- High energy head injury (e.g. pedestrian hit by motor vehicle, fall >1 m or >5 stairs)
- History bleeding or clotting disorder or on anticoagulant therapy
- Difficulty in assessing the patient (e.g. very young, elderly, intoxicated or epileptic) or concern about diagnosis.
- Suspicion of non-accidental injury
- Inadequate supervision at home
- If there is a history of neck pain/neck injury, immobilize the neck and refer to A&E.

If examination is normal
- Warn the patient (+ carer) that s/he may suffer mild headaches, tiredness, dizziness, tinnitus, poor concentration and poor memory for the next few days.
- Advise rest and paracetamol (but not codeine-based analgesics) for the headache.
- Young children can be difficult to assess—sleepiness is common and not a worrying sign as long as the child is rousable.
- Give written head injury information regarding warning signs to trigger reconsultation—drowsiness, severe headache, persistent vomiting, visual disturbance and/or unusual behaviour.

Table 13.5 The Glasgow Coma Scale

Eye opening:	Spontaneous	4
	To voice	3
	To pain	2
	None	1
Best verbal response:	Oriented	5
	Confused	4
	Inappropriate words	3
	Incomprehensive	2
	None	1
Best motor response:	Obeys command	6
	Localizes pain	5
	Withdraw	4
	Flexion	3
	Extension	2
	None	1

Total score = Eye opening + Best verbal + Best motor response scores.

❶ **Watch out for post-concussion syndrome:** seen following even quite minor head injury. Due to neuronal damage.

Features include all or some of:
- Headache
- Dizziness
- Poor concentration
- Fatigue
- Depression
- Memory problems

Treatment is supportive and symptoms usually resolve with time (though can take months or even years).

Further information
NICE Triage, assessment investigation and early management of head injury in infants, children and adults (2003) 🖳 www.nice.org.uk

Advice card for people who have sustained a head injury and/or their carers

We think that it is all right for you to leave the surgery now. We have checked your symptoms and you seem well on the road to recovery.

When you get home it is very unlikely that you will have any further problems. But if any of the following symptoms do return we suggest you get someone to take you to your nearest hospital A&E department as soon as possible:

- Unconsciousness, or lack of full consciousness (for example, problems keeping eyes open)
- Any confusion (not knowing where you are, getting things muddled up)
- Any drowsiness (feeling sleepy)that goes on longer than 1 hour when you would normally be wide awake
- Difficulty waking up
- Any problems understanding or speaking
- Any loss of balance or problems walking
- Any weakness in one or more arms or legs
- Any problems with your eyesight
- Very painful headaches that won't go away
- Any vomiting or getting sick
- Any fits (collapsing or passing out suddenly)
- Clear fluid coming out of your ear or nose
- New bleeding from one or both ears
- New deafness in one or both ears.

Things you shouldn't worry about: you may experience some other symptoms over the next few days which should disappear in the next 2 weeks. These include:

- Mild headache
- Feeling sick (without vomiting)
- Dizziness
- Irritability or bad temper
- Problems concentrating
- Problems with your memory
- Tiredness
- Lack of appetite
- Problems sleeping

If you feel very concerned about any of these symptoms in the first few days, you should come back and see your GP to talk about them.

If these problems do not go away after 2 wk, you should make an appointment to see your GP.

Long-term problems: most people recover quickly from their accident and experience no long-term problems. However, a few people develop problems after weeks or months.

If you start to feel that things are not quite right (for example, memory problems, not feeling yourself), then please contact your doctor as soon as possible so that he/she can make sure you are recovering properly.

Things that will help you get better: if you follow this advice you should get better more quickly and it may help any symptoms you have to go away.

- DO NOT stay at home alone for the first 48 hours after your head injury
- DO make sure you stay within easy reach of a telephone and medical help.
- DO have plenty of rest and avoid stressful situations.
- DO NOT take sleeping pills, sedatives or tranquillizers unless you have checked with your doctor first that it is alright to do so.
- DO NOT play any contact sport (for example, rugby or football) for at least 3 weeks without talking to your doctor first
- DO NOT return to your normal school, college or work activity until you feel you have completely recovered.
- DO NOT drive a car or motorbike, ride a bicycle, or operate machinery unless you feel you have completely recovered

⚠ If you have any effects lasting more than a few days, seek your doctor's opinion about your ability to drive a car or motorbike before driving.

TELEPHONE NUMBER TO CALL IF YOU ARE WORRIED -----------

Reproduced in modified form with permission from NICE *Triage, assessment investigation and early management of head injury in infants, children and adults* (2003) 🖳 www.nice.org.uk

Injury to the face: mostly due to RTAs and violent incidents.
- Document injuries—your notes may be required for legal proceedings.
- Look for other injuries—e.g. airway problems, head injury, neck injury.
- Palpate the face for signs of a fracture—if present refer to maxillofacial surgeons for assessment.
- Check tetanus status.
- Post-traumatic stress disorder is common after facial injury.

⚠ *Neurological assessment* is required if the patient has had a head injury or loss of consciousness. Always look for associated fractures of the zygoma and maxillary bones ('step' deformity in the orbit, dental malocclusion, difficulty opening the jaw, diplopia) and refer urgently to the maxillofacial surgeons if present.

Facial fractures

Nasal fracture: undisplaced nasal fractures can usually be allowed to heal without intervention. X-rays are unhelpful.

Action
- Give adequate analgesia and advise that bruising may be extensive and the nose will feel blocked for 1–2 wk.
- Assessment for permanent deformity can be difficult at the time of the injury due to soft tissue swelling—reassess 7–10 d after injury
- Refer any patient with significant deformity, or if the patient is unhappy with the appearance of their nose, to the ENT department for reduction under GA. Ideally reduction should take place within 1–2 wk (and max. 3 wk) after fracture—so refer promptly.
- Deviation of the nasal septum may not be correctable at the time of manipulation and if symptomatic will need a later submucous resection.

Fractured mandible: a blow to the jaw can cause unilateral or bilateral fractures.

Signs: presents with pain (worse on moving jaw), bruising ± bleeding inside the mouth ± discontinuity of the teeth (displaced fracture) ± numbness of the lower lip (if the inferior dental nerve has been damaged).

Action: Refer for X-ray via A&E.

Fractured zygoma/malar complex: a blow on the cheek may fracture the zygomatic arch in isolation or more usually cause a 'tripod' fracture.

Signs: bony tenderness, flattening of the malar process—best seen from above (may be masked by swelling), epistaxis, subconjunctival haemorrhage extending posteriorly and infraorbital numbness, ± jaw locked.

Action: refer for X-ray via A&E. Advise not to blow nose.

Middle third facial fractures (Le Fort): usually bilateral.

Signs: epistaxis, CSF rhinorrhoea, crepitus on palpation, swelling, open bite and risk of airway compromise.

Action: refer for X-ray via A&E.

'Blow out' fracture of the orbit: 📖 p.174.

Dislocated jaw: presents with pain and the mouth is stuck open—refer for X-ray and reduction via maxillofacial surgeons or A&E.

Knocked out teeth: if there are no other injuries requiring attention, ask the patient to suck the tooth clean, and reinsert the tooth into its socket or store in milk. Send the patient to a dentist.

CSF rhinorrhoea or otorrhoea: clear fluid dripping from the nose or ear after trauma can indicate a fracture and CSF leak. Fluid tests +ve for glucose. It suggests significant trauma—refer to A&E for head injury assessment. Spontaneous healing of the CSF leak is the norm but if it persists refer to neurosurgery for assessment for dural closure.

Septal haematoma: may occur after nasal injury and causes nasal blockage. Presents as a bilateral soft bulging of the septum. Refer urgently to ENT for evacuation to prevent cartilage destruction.

Haematoma of the pinna: usually after trauma (e.g. rugby). Must be evacuated urgently (aspirated via large bore needle or surgically) to prevent necrosis of the cartilage and 'cauliflower' ear—refer to ENT.

Subdural haemorrhage: bleeding is from bridging veins between cortex and venous sinuses, resulting in accumulation of blood between dura and arachnoid. *Causes:* trauma (may be trivial); idiopathic.

Risk factors: age, alcohol, falls, epilepsy, anticoagulant therapy.

Presentation: often insidious and history may go back several weeks:
- Fluctuation of conscious level (35%) and/or sleepiness
- Physical and intellectual slowing and/or personality change
- Headache
- Unsteadiness on feet
- Slowly evolving stroke (e.g. hemiparesis)
- Other symptoms/signs of ↑ICP—VI nerve palsy, papilloedema, dropping pulse, rising BP, pupil changes—constriction first then dilatation.

Differential diagnosis: stroke, cerebral tumour, dementia.

Action: if suspected, admit as a medical emergency for further investigation. Evacuation of clot is possible even in very elderly patients and often results in full recovery.

Extradural haemorrhage: blood accumulates between the dura and bone of the skull. Usually occurs after head injury.

Presentation: deterioration of level of consciousness after head injury that initially produced no loss of consciousness, or after initial post-injury drowsiness has resolved. This 'lucid' interval may last anything from a few hours to a few days. May be accompanied by worsening headache, vomiting, confusion ± focal neurological signs.

Action: if suspected, admit as an emergency for further investigation. Early evacuation of clot carries excellent prognosis. Outlook is less good if coma pre-op.

⊛ **Falls among the elderly**

Falls are a major cause of disability and the leading cause of mortality due to injury in people aged >75 y. Assessment of a patient who has fallen is a common primary care emergency.

Risk factors for falls: recurrence ↑ with number of risk factors:
- ♀:♂ ≈ 2:1 in the over 75s
- ↑ age
- Multiple previous falls
- Disorders of gait or balance
- Visual impairment
- Cognitive impairment
- Low morale/depression
- High level of dependence
- ↓ mobility
- Lower limb weakness or arthritis
- Foot problems
- History of stroke or Parkinson's disease
- Use of psychotropic drugs, sedatives, diuretics or β-blockers
- Alcohol
- Environmental factors, e.g. loose rugs, poor lighting, ice, high winds
- Infection, e.g. pneumonia, UTI

History: deal with the injuries first—ask about pain, loss of function, headache. Ask carers about behaviour.

Examination: check for bruising, loss of function, confusion, BP, pulse, neurology and fundi. Consider hypothermia (📖 p.232) if on the floor any length of time.

Investigate the cause of the fall: *Consider:*
- *Physical problems:* neurological problems (e.g. stroke); visual loss; cardiac abnormalities (e.g. arrythmia, postural hypotension); muscular abnormalities (e.g. steroid induced myopathy); skeletal problems (e.g. osteoarthritis); infection (pneumonia, UTI).
- *Environmental problems:* climbing ladders to do routine maintenance; loose/holed carpets; slippery floor or bath; chair or bed too low.

Management
- *Treat any acute injury.* ❶ Subdural haematoma may take several days or weeks to reveal itself.
- *Perform/refer to a specialist falls service for a falls assessment.*
- *Undertake measures to ↓ risk of falls or damage from falling,* e.g. review medication, remove hazards (loose carpets etc.).

Refer to A&E if
- Significant head injury (📖 p.222)
- Any suspicion of fracture
- Any other significant injury, e.g. lacerations.

Admit to the acute medical team or elderly care team if:
- Cause of the fall was an acute medical problem, e.g. stroke
- The patient is unable to cope at home.

Refer to the specialist elderly care team if:
- The cause of recurrent falls remains unclear
- The patient or carer are worried about the possibility of further falls *or*
- There is doubt about whether the patient can cope in their current social circumstances.

Box 13.2 Consequences of falling

- 20% who experience a fall will incur an injury requiring acute medical attention—though <1:10 falls result in a fracture (mainly Colles' and fractured neck of femur).
- Even if uninjured, older people might not be able to get up off the floor without help. The result may be a prolonged period of lying on the floor until help arrives. Apart from the indignity and helplessness this generates, secondary problems, e.g. pneumonia, pressure sores, hypothermia, UTI and dehydration may follow.
- Any fall may seriously undermine an elderly person's confidence and make him/her (and his/her relatives/carers) worry about the possibility of recurrence. As a result, he/she may restrict activities becoming less fit and more dependent on others.

⊛ **Scalds and burns**

Assess
- Cause, size and thickness of the burn.
- Use the 'rule of nines' to estimate the extent of the burn (Box 13.3).
- Partial thickness burns are red, painful and blistered, full thickness burns are painless and white or grey.
- Always consider non-accidental injury in children—🕮 p.126.

⚠ **Action**
- Remove clothing from the affected area and place under cold running water for >10 min or until pain is relieved.
- Do not burst blisters.
- Prescribe/give analgesia.
- Refer all but the smallest (<5%) partial thickness burns for assessment in A&E.
- Refer all electrical burns for assessment in A&E.
- Refer all chemical burns for assessment in A&E unless burn area is minimal and pain-free.
- Consider referral to A&E for smoke inhalation.

If managing the burn in the community:
- Check tetanus immunity and give immunization ± prophylaxis as necessary—🕮 p.215.
- Apply silver sulfadiazine cream (flamazine) or vaseline impregnated gauze and non-adherent dressings and review for healing and infection every 1–2 d.
- Cover burns on hands in flamazine and place in a plastic bag—elevate the hand in a sling and encourage finger movement.
- Refer if burns are not healed in 10–12 d.

Prevention of scalds and burns
- Prevention through public education is important.
- Children often sustain burns by pulling on the flex of boiling kettles or irons, pulling on saucepan handles or climbing onto hot cookers.
- Refer any children who have sustained accidental burns to the health visitor for follow-up.

Smoke inhalation
- Refer all patients who have potentially inhaled smoke for assessment—a seemingly well patient can deteriorate later.
- Smoke can cause thermal injury, carbon monoxide poisoning and cyanide poisoning.
- Airway problems occur due to thermal and chemical damage to the airways causing oedema—suspect if singed nasal hairs, a sore throat or a hoarse voice.
- Carbon monoxide poisoning may result in the classic cherry-red mucosa—but this may be absent.
- Cyanide poisoning is commonly due to smouldering plastics and causes dizziness, headaches and seizures.

Sunburn: susceptibility depends on skin type.
- Tingling is followed 2–12 h later by erythema. Redness is maximal at 24 h and fades over 2–3 d. Desquamation and pigmentation follow.
- Severe sunburn may cause blistering, pain and systemic upset. Treatment is symptomatic with calamine lotion prn (some advocate application of vinegar).and paracetamol for pain
- Rarely dressings are required for blisters or, in severe cases, hospital admission for fluid management
- Predisposes to skin cancer and photoageing.

The sun safety code: take care not to burn in the sun
- Cover up with loose cool clothing, a hat and sun glasses
- If swimming outdoors or on the beach, dress in a UV protective sunsuit. When out of the water, add a T-shirt, sun glasses and sun hat.
- Seek shade during the hottest part of the day
- Apply sunscreen (≥SPF 25) on sun-exposed parts of the body.

Box 13.3 Rule of Nines: ignore areas of erythema only

Palm	1%
Arm (all over)	9%
Leg (all over)	18% (14% children)
Front	18%
Back	18%
Head (all over)	9% (14% children)
Genitals	1%

⚠ The Rule of Nines is inaccurate for children <10 y. For children and for small burns, estimate the extent of the burn by comparison with the area of the patient's hand. The area of the fingers and palm ≈ 1% total body surface area burn.

Burns in special situations

Chemical burns
- Usually caused by strong acids or alkalis.
- Wear gloves to remove contaminated clothing.
- Irrigate with cold running water for ≥20 min.
- Do not attempt to neutralize the chemical—this can exacerbate injury by producing heat.
- Refer all burns to A&E unless the burn area is minimal and pain free.

Electric shock
- Causes thermal tissue injury and direct injury due to the electric current passing through the tissue.
- Skin burns may be seen at the entry and exit site of the current.
- Muscle damage can be severe with minimal skin injury.
- Cardiac damage may occur and rhabdomyolysis can → renal failure.
- Refer all patients for specialist management.

☼ / ⊛ Environmental emergencies

Sunburn: 📖 p.231.

Hypothermia: defined as a core temperature of <35°C.

Causes
- Not feeling the cold, e.g. neuropathy, confusion, dementia
- Inadequate heat in the home, e.g. poor housing, poverty
- Immobility
- Hypothyroidism
- Diabetes
- ↑ heat loss, e.g. psoriasis, erythroderma
- Inadequate protection from the cold, e.g. unsuitable clothing while doing outdoor sports
- Alcohol
- Drugs—antipsychotics, antidepressants, barbiturates, tranquilizers—may lower the level of consciousness and ↓ ability to shiver
- Falls—may remain still and cold until discovered
- Unconsciousness, e.g. overdose, stroke.

Presentation
- Skin pale cold to touch
- Puffy-face
- Listlessness, drowsiness and/or confusion.

When severe
- ↓ breathing—slow and shallow
- ↓ pulse volume—faint and irregular
- Stiff muscles
- Loss of consciousness.

Investigation
- Rectal temperature on low-reading thermometer <35°C
- ECG—'J' wave on the end of the QRS complex.

Action
- Remove from the cold environment
- Wrap in blankets—including head
- Do not use direct heat (e.g. hot water bottles) as this can cause rapid fluid shifts and potentially fatal pulmonary oedema
- Transfer to hospital
- Consider the cause of the incident and liaise with the hospital, primary healthcare team and social services to prevent recurrence in the future.

Heat stroke and heat exhaustion: exercising in excessive heat leads to dehydration, salt depletion and metabolite accumulation.

Signs: headache, nausea, confusion, incoordination, cramps, weakness, dizziness, malaise.

Treatment: rest, fluid and salt replacement. Admission for IV fluids and supportive measures in severe cases.

Drowning: most common in drunk adults and children poorly supervised around water. Children can drown in a few centimetres of water.

⚠ *Action*

- Call for help
- Start basic life support (**A**irway, **B**reathing, **C**irculation)—
  📖 p.18 (adults); 📖 p.24 (children)

⚠ Attempted resuscitation of a seemingly dead child is worthwhile as cooling ↓ metabolic rate and recovery can occur after prolonged immersion.

Acute altitude sickness: potentially fatal complication of rapidly climbing to altitudes >8000 feet. 2 main forms:
- Pulmonary oedema
- Cerebral oedema.

Presentation: fatigue, headache, dizziness, nausea/loss of appetite, breathlessness, palpitations, insomnia.

Management: oxygen therapy and descent to a lower altitude

Prevention: gradual ascent.

◉ /⌂ **Domestic violence**

Used to describe physical, emotional and mental abuse of women by male partners. Affects ~1:4 women—the most common form of interpersonal crime. 60%—current partner; 21%—former partners. ½ suffer >1 attack. $^1/_3$ have been attacked repeatedly.

General practice is often the first place in which women seek formal help but only ¼ actually reveal they have been beaten. Without appropriate intervention, violence continues and often ↑ in frequency and severity. By the time the woman's injuries are visible, violence may be a long-established pattern. On average, a woman will be assaulted 35 times before reporting it to police.

Effects: high incidence of psychiatric disorders, particularly depression, and self-damaging behaviours including drug and alcohol abuse, suicide and parasuicide.

Factors preventing the woman leaving the abusive situation

- Loss of self-esteem makes women think they are to blame
- Fear of partner
- Disruption of the family and children's relationship with their father
- Loss of intimate relationship with partner
- Fall in income
- Risk of homelessness
- Fear of the unknown.

Guidelines for care

- Consider the possibility of domestic violence—ask directly.
- Emphasize confidentiality.
- Document—accurate, clear documentation, over time at successive consultations, may provide cumulative evidence of abuse, and is essential for use as evidence in court, should the need arise.
- Assess the present situation—Gather as much information as possible.
- Provide information and offer help in making contact with other agencies.
- Devise a safety plan—give the 'phone number of local women's refuge; advise to keep some money and important financial and legal documents hidden in a safe place in case of emergency; help plan an escape route in case of emergency.

❶ Do not pressurize women into any course of action. If the patient decides to return to the violent situation, she will not forget the information and support given. In time this might give her the confidence and back up she needs to break out of her situation.

⚠ If children are likely to be at risk you have a duty to inform social services or police, preferably with the patient's consent

Elder abuse: defined as: 'A single or repeated act or lack of appropriate action, occurring within any relationship where there is an expectation of trust, which causes harm or distress to an older person'.

Older people may report the abuse but often do not. May take several forms which may coexist:

- *Physical,* e.g. cuts, bruises, unexplained fractures, dehydration/ malnourishment with no medical explanation, burns
- *Psychological,* e.g. unusual behaviour, unexplained fear, appears helpless or withdrawn
- *Financial,* e.g. removal of funds by carers, new will in favour of carer
- *Sexual,* e.g. unexplained bruising, vaginal or anal bleeding, genital infections
- *Neglect,* e.g. malnourished, dehydrated, poor personal hygiene, late requests for medical attention.

Prevalence (in own home): physical abuse, 2%; verbal abuse, 5%; financial abuse, 2%.

Signs: inconsistent story from patient and carer, inconsistencies on examination; fear in presence of carer; frequent attendance at A&E; frequent requests for GP visits; carer avoiding GP.

Management: talk through the situation with the patient, carer and other services involved in care. Assess the level of risk. Consider admission to a place of safety—contact social services and/or police as necessary; seek advice from Action on Elder Abuse.

Further information

Department of Health. Domestic violence: A resource manual for health care professionals. Available from 🖳 www.dh.gov.uk

Home office: 🖳 www.homeoffice.gov.uk/crime-victims/reducing-crime/domestic-violence

RCGP: Heath I. Domestic violence. 🖳 www.rcgp.org.uk

BMJ: Ramsay J. et al. Should health professionals screen women for domestic violence? Systematic review. BMJ 2002: 325; 314

Useful contacts

Womens' aid: ☎ 0808 2000 247 🖳 www.womensaid.org.uk

Action on elder abuse ☎ 0808 808 8141 🖳 www.elderabuse.org.uk

Police domestic violence units ☎ 0845 045 45 45

Local authority social services departments

Local authority housing departments

---

❶ Domestic violence may start or escalate in pregnancy—estimated prevalence is 17%. It ↑ risk of preterm birth, antepartum haemorrhage and perinatal mortality. Ask routinely about domestic violence as part of usual antenatal care.

⌂/☺ **Assault and rape**

Victims of crime: victims need treatment of injuries and emotional support. Record information carefully as it may be needed for legal cases. Note the date, time and place of the event. Record injuries in detail (physical and psychological)—including measuring the size of lacerations and bruises. Arrange for photos to be taken (police may arrange this). Encourage reporting of the incident to the police (the patient will not be eligible for criminal injury compensation if it is not reported). Give patient details of local victim support groups. If the patient's safety is an issue, contact the duty social worker for a place of safety.

Rape and indecent assault: if a patient reports rape or indecent assault and is willing to report the matter to the police, do not examine her/him. The case against the assailant could be won or lost on the basis of evidence gained by examination of an alleged victim so it is best done by a doctor trained and experienced in such work. If the patient will not report the matter to the police, other options open to the woman are self-presentation to a genitourinary medicine clinic or sexual assault treatment centre (SATC).

If assessing a woman in general practice, take a full history and note LMP, contraception, sexual history. Make a note of any injuries and take photographs if possible and appropriate. Do not insist on examination if the patient is unwilling. Ensure a chaperone is present if any examination is attempted. Discuss the need for emergency contraception, prophylactic antibiotics (e.g. ciprofloxacin 250 mg po stat), blood tests at 3 mo to exclude transmission of syphilis and 3–6 mo for exclusion of seroconversion for HIV.

If at high risk for HIV transmission refer to A&E for consideration of prophylaxis (📖 p.157). Discuss the need for counselling and inform the patient about the victim support scheme and rape crisis centres. Arrange follow-up in 2–3 wk.

Criminal Injuries compensation: for victims of violent crimes—even if the attacker is not identified. Compensation is paid for the injury, loss of earnings and expenses. Claim by contacting the Criminal injuries Compensation Authority, Tay House, 300 Bath Street, Glasgow G2 4LN ☎ 0800 358 3601 🖥 www.cica.gov.uk

Post-traumatic stress disorder (PTSD): 📖 p.34. 23% assault victims and 80% rape victims develop PTSD. ♀:♂ ≈ 2:1.

Child abuse: 📖 p.126.

Elder abuse: 📖 p.235.

Domestic violence: 📖 p.234.

Further information

Treating victims of crime Guidelines for health professionals. Victim support (National office—Cranmer House, 39 Brixton road, London SW9 6DZ. ☎ 020 7735 9166 🖥 www.victimsupport.org)

Patient information and support

Victim support ☎ 0845 3030 900; 🖳 www.victimsupport.org
Rape crisis UK and Ireland 🖳 www.rapecrisis.org.uk
Survivors UK provides resources for men who have experienced any form of sexual violence
☎ 0845 122 1201 🖳 www.survivorsuk.org

Chapter 14

Dermatology and palliative care emergencies

👁 Skin emergencies

Erythroderma: Inflammatory dermatosis affecting >90% skin surface. Rare, but systemic effects are potentially fatal. ♂:♀ ≈ 2:1. Typical patient is middle aged or elderly. Patchy erythema becomes universal in <48 h. Accompanied by fever, shivering and malaise. 2–6d later scaling appears. The skin is hot, red, itchy, dry, thickened and feels tight. Hair and nails may be shed.

Cause: eczema (40%); psoriasis (25%); lymphoma (15%); drug eruption (10%); other skin disease (2%); unknown (8%).

Management: admit as an acute medical emergency.

Scalded skin syndrome: acute toxic illness usually of infants. Characterized by shedding of sheets of skin. May follow impetigo.

Management: emergency paediatric admission. Requires IV antibiotics.

Erysipelas and cellulitis: acute infection of the dermis usually affecting the face or lower leg.

Presentation
- May be preceded by fever ± 'flu-like' symptoms.
- Presents with a painful, reddened area with a well-defined edge ± local swelling ± blistering.
- There may be an obvious entry wound.

Management: oral penicillin V or erythromycin 250–500 mg qds for 7–14 d. Severe infections may require hospital admission for IV antibiotics. Recurrent infections (>2 episodes at 1 site) require prophylactic long-term penicillin (e.g. penicillin V od or bd) and attention to potential entry portals (e.g. tinea pedis).

Complications: lymphangitis ± permanent damage to lymph drainage; glomerulonephritis; guttate psoriasis.

Necrotizing fasciitis: acute and serious infection. Usually occurs in otherwise healthy individuals after surgery or trauma (may be minor). Ill-defined erythema associated with high fever. Rapidly becomes necrotic.

Management: emergency admission for IV antibiotics ± surgical debridement.

Paronychia, boils and carbuncles: infection of hair follicles is usually with *Staphylococcus aureus*. Predisposing factors include DM, obesity and immunosuppression.

- *Acute paronychia:* infection of the skin and soft tissue of nail fold, most commonly caused by *Staphylococcus aureus*. Often originates from a break in the skin as a result of minor trauma, e.g. nail biting. Skin and soft tissue of the nail fold are red, hot, and tender; nail may appear discoloured/distorted.
- *Boil:* hard, tender, red nodule surrounding a hair follicle becoming larger and fluctuant after several days. May discharge pus before healing and leave a scar

- *Carbuncle*: swollen, painful area discharging pus from several points. Occurs when a group of hair follicles become deeply infected. May be associated with fever ± malaise.

Management
- Apply moist heat to relieve discomfort, help localize the infection, and promote drainage.
- If there is associated fever, surrounding cellulitis or the lesion is on the face treat with oral antibiotics, e.g. flucloxacillin or erythromycin 250–500 mg qds.
- If lesion is large, painful and fluctuant consider admission for incision and drainage (young child, uncooperative child, boil in a sensitive area, e.g. genital region, face, neck, axilla, breast area). Do not attempt incision and drainage in the surgery if you are not confident. After incision and drainage treat with oral antibiotics until inflammation resolves.
- If the lesion is not settling with primary care treatment, admit.

Staphylococcal whitlow (felon): infection involving the bulbous distal pulp of the finger following trauma or extension from an acute paronychia. Rapid onset of erythema, swelling and exquisite tenderness of the finger bulb. *Differential diagnosis:* herpetic whitlow. *Management:* Admit for drainage and antibiotics.

Perianal haematoma (thrombosed external pile): due to a ruptured superficial perianal vein → a subcutaneous haematoma. Presents with sudden onset of severe perianal pain. A tender, 2–4 mm 'dark blue berry' under the skin adjacent to the anus is visible. Treat with analgesia. Settles spontaneously over ~ 1 wk If the haematoma is <1 d old, it can be evacuated via a small incision under LA.

Perianal abscess: usually caused by infection arising in a perianal gland. Tends to lie between the internal and external sphincters and points towards the skin at the anal margin. May affect patients of any age and presents with gradual onset of perianal pain, which becomes throbbing and severe; defecation and sitting are painful—characteristically patients sit with one buttock raised off the chair. Examination may reveal the abscess in the skin next to the anus. Refer as an acute surgical emergency for drainage.

⊛ / 🔔 **Emergencies in palliative care**

Some acute events in advanced disease must be treated as an emergency. While unnecessary hospital admission may cause distress for patients/carers, missed emergency treatment of reversible conditions can be disastrous.

Questions to ask when managing emergencies
- What is the problem?
- Can it be reversed?
- What effect will reversal have on this patient's overall condition?
- Could active treatment maintain/improve this patient's quality of life?
- What do you think is the 'right' thing to do?
- What does the patient want?
- What do the carers want?

Table 14.1 Emergencies in advanced disease

Condition	Emergency management
Hypercalcaemia	Depending on the general state of the patient, make a decision whether to treat the hypercalcaemia or not.
	If a decision is made not to treat: provide symptom control and don't check the serum calcium again.
	Active treatment: depends on level of symptoms and Ca^{2+}:
	• asymptomatic patient with corrected calcium <3 mmol/l—monitor
	• symptomatic and/or corrected calcium >3 mmol/l—arrange treatment with pamidronate via oncologist/palliative care team immediately.
Bone fracture	Give analgesia
	Unless in a very terminal state, confirm the fracture on X-ray and refer to orthopaedics or radiotherapy urgently for consideration of fixation (long bones, wrist, neck of femur) and/or radiotherapy (rib fractures, vertebral fractures).
Massive bleeding Haematuria Haemoptysis GI bleeding Wounds	Make a decision whether the cause of the bleed is treatable or a terminal event.
	Active treatment: call for emergency ambulance support. Lie flat. Gain IV access and give IV fluids if available.
	No active treatment: stay with the patient, give sedative medication (e.g. midazolam 10–40 mg s/cut or IM or diazepam 10–20 mg pr. Support the carers. Consider diamorphine 2–10 mg s/cut if the patient is in pain.
Acute breathlessness 📖 p.78	*Consider reversible causes*: anaemia, pneumonia, pleural effusion, exacerbation of COPD, heart failure, PE, superior vena cava obstruction
	Palliative measures: morphine 2.5–5 mg prn (or ↑ background opioid dose by 30–50%) or consider diamorphine/morphine syringe driver with midazolam 5–10 mg over 24 h.

Table 14.1 (contd.)

Condition	Emergency management
Spinal cord compression	Presents with back pain worse on movement and neurological symptoms, e.g. constipation, weak legs, incontinence of urine.
	Prompt treatment (<24–48 h from 1st neurological symptoms) is needed if there is any hope of restoring function. Treat with oral dexamethasone 16 mg/d and refer urgently for radiotherapy unless in final stages of disease.
Pain	*Breakthrough of pre-existing, opioid responsive pain:* give a stat dose of opioid = 1/6th total opioid dose in the last 24 h. Acts in <30 min. Repeat if ineffective.
	To convert 24 h doses:
	• Oral morphine 90 mg = s/cut diamorphine 30 mg (3:1)
	• Oral morphine 90 mg = s/cut morphine 45 mg (2:1)
	• Fentanyl '25' patch = s/cut diamorphine 30 mg
Opioid overdosage	If respiratory rate ≥8/min and patient is easily rousable and not cyanosed—review if condition worsens. Consider reducing or omitting the next regular dose of opioid.
	If respiratory rate <8/min, and/or the patient is barely rousable/unconscious and/or cyanosed dilute a standard ampoule containing naloxone 400 mcgm to 10 ml with sodium chloride 0.9%. Administer 0.5 ml (20 mcgm) IV every 2 min until respiratory status is satisfactory. If respiratory function does not improve in 10 min, question diagnosis.
	❶ Further boluses may be necessary once respiratory function improves as naloxone is shorter acting than morphine.
Fitting	Ensure the airway is clear and turn the patient into the recovery position. Prevent onlookers from restraining the fitting patient
	Treat fitting with diazepam 5–10 mg IV or pr.
	If >1 seizure without the patient regaining consciousness *or* fitting continues >20 min repeat diazepam every 15 min until fitting is controlled. Unless in a very terminal condition admit.
	Support carers
	Consider checking BM. Depending on clinical state, consider referral for further investigation if first fit.
Terminal restlessness/ agitation	*Causes:* pain/discomfort, myoclonic jerks 2° to opioid toxicity, biochemical causes (e.g. ↑ Ca^{2+}, uraemia), psychological/ spiritual distress.
	Management:
	• Treat reversible causes, e.g. catheterization for retention, hyoscine to dry up secretions
	• If still restless, treat with a sedative. This does NOT shorten life but makes the patient and any relatives in attendance more comfortable.
	Suitable drugs: haloperidol 1–3 mg tds po; diazepam 2–10 mg tds po, midazolam (10–100 mg/24 h via syringe driver or 5 mg stat) or levomepromazine (12.5–50 mg/24 h via syringe driver or 6.25 mg stat).

Psychiatric emergencies

🔔 Acute panic attacks

Common primary care emergency that can be difficult to manage.

Features: fear, terror and feeling of impending doom accompanied by some or all of the following:
- Palpitations
- Shortness of breath
- Choking sensation
- Dizziness
- Paraesthesiae
- Chest pain/discomfort
- Sweating
- Carpopedal spasm.

Differential diagnosis
- Dysrhythmia
- Asthma
- Anaphylaxis
- Thyrotoxicosis
- Temporal lobe epilepsy
- Hypoglycaemia
- Phaeochromocytoma (very rare).

Action
Talking down: explain the nature of the symptoms to the patient:
- Racing of the heart is due to adrenaline produced by the panic
- Paraesthesiae and feelings of dizziness are due to overbreathing due to panic
- Count breaths in and out gently slowing breathing rate.

Rebreathing techniques
- Place a paper bag over the patient's mouth and ask him to breath in and out through the mouth.
- A connected but not switched on O_2 mask or nebulizer mask is an alternative in the surgery.
- This raises the partial pressure of CO_2 in the blood and symptoms due to low CO_2 (e.g. tetany, paraesthesiae, dizziness) resolve. This demonstrates the link between hyperventilation and the symptoms too.

Propranolol: 10–20 mg stat may be helpful—DON'T USE for asthmatics or patients with heart failure or on verapamil.

Self-help for patients

One way of tackling panic attacks is to look at the way you talk to yourself, especially during times of stress and pressure. Panic attacks often begin or escalate when you tell yourself scary things, like 'I feel light-headed ... I'm about to faint!' or 'I'm trapped in this traffic jam and something terrible is gonna happen!' or 'If I go outside, I'll freak out.' These are called 'negative predictions' and they have a strong influence on the way your body feels. If you're mentally predicting a disaster, your body's alarm response goes off and the 'fight–flight response' kicks in.

To combat this, try to focus on calming, positive thoughts, like 'I'm learning to deal with panicky feelings and I know that people overcome panic all the time' or 'This will pass quickly, and I can help myself by concentrating on my breathing and imagining a relaxing place' or 'These feelings are uncomfortable, but they won't last forever.'

Remind yourself of these FACTS about panic attacks:
- A panic attack cannot cause heart failure or a heart attack.
- A panic attack cannot cause you to stop breathing.
- A panic attack cannot cause you to faint.
- A panic attack cannot cause you to 'go crazy.'
- A panic attack cannot cause you to lose control of yourself.

If it's too hard to think calming thoughts when you're having a panic attack, find ways to distract yourself. Some people do this by talking to other people when they feel the panic coming on. Others prefer to exercise or work on a detailed project or hobby. Changing scenery can sometimes be helpful, too, but it's important not to get into a pattern of avoiding necessary daily tasks. If you notice that you're regularly avoiding things like driving, going shopping, going to work, or taking public transport, it's probably time to get some professional help.

Slow, abdominal breathing (6 breaths per minute) has been shown to stop panic attacks. Learning slow abdominal breathing can be quite difficult and people who have panic attacks are almost always chest breathers. Practice abdominal breathing (moving upper part of tummy to breath rather than chest wall) when relaxed at home. If you can learn to breathe slowly with your diaphragm, you will not panic!

Cut down on alcohol and caffeine—these can make panic attacks worse. Try relaxation techniques (such as yoga) and exercise regularly—both can help reduce the number of panic attacks people have.

Information and support for patients

Royal College of Psychiatrists: Patient information sheets 🖳 www.rcpsych.ac.uk
No more panic 🖳 www.nomorepanic.co.uk

⊛ / 🔔 Poisoning or overdose

On receiving the call for assistance

- Try to establish what has happened—substances involved, ongoing dangers, state of the patient.
- Advise the caller to stay with the patient until you arrive.
- If the patient is unconscious, arrange for an ambulance to meet you at the scene.
- Arrange for the patient to be removed from any source of danger, e.g. contaminated clothing or inhaled gases. DO NOT put yourself or anyone else in danger attempting to do this. If necessary call the fire brigade , who have protective clothing and equipment, to help remove a patient from a dangerous environment.

Assessment of the unconscious patient

Assess the need for basic life support

- Airway patent?
- Breathing satisfactory?
- Circulation adequate?

Resuscitation (📖 p.18–29) takes priority over everything else.

Additionally

- If breathing is depressed and opioid overdose is a possibility give naloxone 0.4–2 mg IV every 2–3 min to a maximum of 10 mg (*Child* – 10 mcgm/kg and then, if no response, 100 mcgm/kg).
- Check BM—if low give 50–250 ml 10% glucose IV in 50 ml aliquots.

General examination

- BP
- Pulse
- Temperature
- Level of coma (📖 p.42)
- Pupil responses
- Evidence of IV drug abuse
- Obvious injury

❶ The coma may not be due to poisoning/overdose.

If unconscious, turn into the recovery position: 📖 p.30. Check no contra-indications first, e.g. spinal injury

Note down any information about the exposure

- *Product name:* as much detail as possible—if unidentified tablets, see if any are left and send them to the hospital in their own container (if there is one) with the patient.
- *Time of the incident*
- *Duration of exposure/amount ingested*
- *Route of exposure*—swallowed, inhaled, injected etc.
- *Whether intentional or accidental*
- *Take a general history from any attendant*—medical history, current medication, substance abuse, alcohol, social circumstances.

Assessment of the conscious patient

- Note down any information about the exposure as for the unconscious patient.
- Record symptoms the patient is experiencing as a result of exposure.
- Examine—pulse, BP, temperature (if necessary), level of consciousness or confusion, evidence of IV drug abuse, any injuries.
- If non-accidental exposure assess suicidal intent (📖 p.251).
- Take a general history from the patient and/or any attendant—medical history, current medication, substance abuse, alcohol, social circumstances.

Children: peak incidence of accidental poisoning is at 2 y—mainly household substances, prescribed or OTC drugs, or plants. Teenagers may take deliberate overdoses—especially of OTC medication, e.g. paracetamol.

⚠ Poisoning can be a form of non-accidental injury (📖 p.126).

Action

Consider admission if

- The patient's clinical condition warrants it: unconsciousness, respiratory depression, etc.
- The exposure warrants admission for treatment or observation:
  - symptomatic poisoning: admit to hospital
  - agents with delayed action: aspirin, iron, paracetamol, tricyclic antidepressants, Lomotil (co-phenotrope), paraquat and modified release preparations. Admit to hospital even if the patient seems well.
  - other agents: consult poisons information.
- You judge there is serious suicidal intent (📖 p.251) or the patient has another psychiatric condition which warrants acute admission.
- There is a lack of social support.

Poisons information

UK National Poisons Information Service ☎ 0870 600 6266 (Ireland: (01) 809 2566)
TOXBASE poisons database 🖳 www.spib.axl.co.uk

⊛ / ⌂ Suicide and deliberate self-harm

❶ People who have self-harmed should be treated with the same care respect and privacy as any other patient.

Deliberate self-harm (DSH): deliberate non-fatal act committed in the knowledge that it was potentially harmful and, in the case of drug overdose, that the amount taken was excessive. 90% DSH is due to self-poisoning and it accounts for 20% of admissions to general medical wards—the most frequent reason for admission for young ♀ patients. Paracetamol or aspirin are the most common drugs used. Self-harm is often aimed at changing a situation (e.g. to get a boyfriend back), communication of distress ('cry for help'), a sign of emotional distress or may be a failed genuine suicide attempt.

Action: calls to patients who have deliberately self-harmed themselves, are threatening suicide or if relatives are worried about suicide risk are common primary care emergencies.
- Algorithm for assessment of patients who have deliberately self-harmed, threatened or attempted suicide—Figure 15.1, 🕮 p.252
- Algorithm for management of patients who have deliberately self-harmed, threatened or attempted suicide—Figure 15.2, 🕮 p.253.

Compulsory admission under the Mental Health Act: 🕮 p.258.

Suicide prevention: Our Healthier Nation set a target to ↓ death by suicide by 17% by 2010. GPs play a crucial role in achieving this target. The UK suicide rate is 1:6000 and the average GP will have 10–15 patients who commit suicide during a career in general practice. In ♂ <35y suicide is now the most common cause of death. The National Suicide Prevention Strategy for England sets out 6 goals and objectives:
- To ↓ risk in key high-risk groups
- To promote mental well-being in the wider population
- To ↓ availability and lethality of suicide methods
- To improve reporting of suicidal behaviour in the community
- To promote research on suicide and suicide prevention
- To improve monitoring of progress towards the Saving Lives: Our Healthier Nation target to ↓ suicide.

Support of those bereaved through suicide: those bereaved through suicide face special problems. Give as much support as possible, try to ↓ stigma, suggest self-help groups and/or counselling.

Further information

NICE Self-harm: The short-term physical and psychological management and secondary prevention of self-harm in primary and secondary care (2004) 🖳 www.nice.org.uk
DoH National Suicide Prevention Strategy for England (2002) 🖳 www.dh.gov.uk

Useful questions for assessing suicidal ideas and plans

- Do you feel you have a future?
- Do you feel that life's not worth living?
- Do you ever feel completely hopeless?
- Do you ever feel you'd be better off dead and away from it all?
- Have you ever made any plans to end your life (if drug overdose—have you handled the tablets)?
- Have you ever made an attempt to take your own life?—if so, was there a final act, e.g. suicide note?
- What prevents you doing it?
- Have you made any arrangements for your affairs after your death?

What can be done in primary care to prevent suicide?

- Early recognition, assessment and treatment of those likely to attempt suicide is key to the primary care role—many visit their GP just weeks before suicide.
- Restrict access to lethal agents, e.g. avoid tricyclic antidepressants and monitor repeat prescriptions of antidepressants carefully.
- Plan follow-up care for those discharged from psychiatric hospital.

Information and support for patients and relatives

Self injury and related issues (SIARI) 🖳 www.siari.co.uk
Samaritans 24 h emotional support via telephone ☎ 08457 909 090 🖳 www.samaritans.org.uk
Survivors of bereavement by suicide ☎ 0870 241 3337 🖳 www.uk-sobs.org.uk

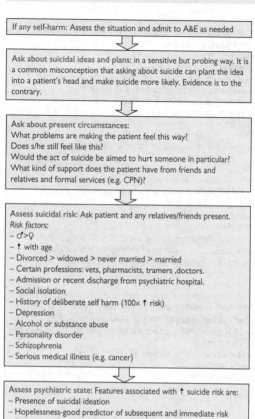

If any self-harm: Assess the situation and admit to A&E as needed

Ask about suicidal ideas and plans: in a sensitive but probing way. It is a common misconception that asking about suicide can plant the idea into a patient's head and make suicide more likely. Evidence is to the contrary.

Ask about present circumstances:
What problems are making the patient feel this way?
Does s/he still feel like this?
Would the act of suicide be aimed to hurt someone in particular?
What kind of support does the patient have from friends and relatives and formal services (e.g. CPN)?

Assess suicidal risk: Ask patient and any relatives/friends present.
Risk factors:
– ♂>♀
– ↑ with age
– Divorced > widowed > never married > married
– Certain professions: vets, pharmacists, tramers ,doctors.
– Admission or recent discharge from psychiatric hospital.
– Social isolation
– History of deliberate self harm (100× ↑ risk)
– Depression
– Alcohol or substance abuse
– Personality disorder
– Schizophrenia
– Serious medical illness (e.g. cancer)

Assess psychiatric state: Features associated with ↑ suicide risk are:
– Presence of suicidal ideation
– Hopelessness-good predictor of subsequent and immediate risk
– Depression
– Agitation
– Early schizophrenia with retained insight—especially young patients who see their ambitions restricted
– Presence of delusions of control, poverty and/or guilt.

Fig. 15.1 Assessment of patients who have deliberately self harmed, threatened or attempted suicide.

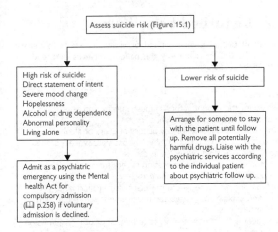

Fig. 15.2 Management of patients who have deliberately self harmed, threatened or attempted suicide.

:Ö: / ⊗ Disturbed behaviour

When a patient becomes very agitated or violent or starts to behave oddly, the GP is usually called—by the patient, relatives or friends or police attending the disturbance.

Assessment

- Before seeing the patient gather as much information as possible from notes, relatives—even neighbours.
- Ask the patient and family for any history of drugs or alcohol excess.
- Listen to the patient and talk calmly—choose your words carefully.
- Try to look for organic causes—this can be difficult in the heat of the moment—physical examination except from a distance may be impossible. Don't put yourself at risk.
- Suspect an organic cause where there are visual hallucinations.
- Discuss and explain your suggested management with the patient and any attendants.
- If the patient is an immediate danger to himself or others, admission is warranted.
- If the cause of the behaviour is unclear, admission for investigation is needed.
- Instigate management of treatable causes identified, e.g. admit if MI suspected; treat UTI.
- Consider sedation to cover the period before admission or to alleviate symptoms if admission is inappropriate.

Causes of disturbed behaviour

- *Physical illness causing acute confusional state*—infection (e.g. UTI, chest infection); hypoglycaemia; hypoxia; head injury; epilepsy
- *Drugs*—alcohol (or alcohol withdrawal); prescribed drugs (e.g. steroid psychosis); illicit drugs (e.g. amphetamines).
- *Psychiatric illness*—schizophrenia; mania; anxiety/depression; dementia; personality disorder (e.g. attention-seeking; uncontrolled anger).

Acute management: after assessing the problem, decide if hospitalization is required and whether this can be done on a voluntary or involuntary basis.

Suitable drugs to use for sedation

- *Oral:* diazepam 5–10 mg po or lorazepam 1 mg po/s/ling; chlorpromazine 50–100 mg po.
- *Intramuscular:* chlorpromazine 50 mg; haloperidol 1–3 mg.

❶ *Avoid sedating* patients with COPD, epilepsy or if the patient has been taking illicit drugs, barbiturates or alcohol.

Compulsory admission under the Mental health Act: 🕮 p.258.

⚠ **Look after your own safety**
- If the patient is known to be violent, get back up from the police before entering the situation.
- Tell someone you are going in and when to expect an 'exit' call. Advise them to call for help if that call is not made.
- Do not put yourself in a vulnerable situation—sit where there is a clear, unimpeded exit route.
- Do not make the patient feel trapped.
- Do not try to restrain the patient.

⚠ **Acute dystonia:** can occur soon after giving phenothiazines or butyophenones. *Signs:*
- torticollis
- tongue protrusion
- grimacing
- opisthotonus.

Dystonia can be relieved with IM procyclidine 5–10 mg (repeated prn after 20 min to a maximum dose of 20 mg).

⊛ Acute confusional states (delirium)

Common condition seen in general practice—particularly among elderly patients. May occur de novo or be superimposed upon chronic confusion of dementia resulting in sudden worsening of cognition.

Presentation

- Global cognitive deficit with onset over hours/days
- Fluctuating conscious level—typically worse at night/late afternoon
- Impaired memory—on recovery amnesia of the events is usual
- Disorientation in time and place
- Odd behaviour—may be underactive, drowsy and/or withdrawn *or* hyperactive and agitated
- Disordered thinking—often slow and muddled ± delusions (e.g. accuse relatives of taking things)
- Disturbed perceptions—hallucinations (particularly visual) are common
- Mood swings.

Examination: can be difficult. If possible do a thorough general physical examination to exclude treatable causes.

Possible causes: Table 15.1.

Differential diagnosis

- Deafness: may appear confused
- Dementia: longer history and lack of fluctuations in conscious level—in practice may be difficult to distinguish especially if you come across a patient who is alone and can give no history
- Primary mental illness, e.g. schizophrenia; anxiety state.

Management: is aimed at treating all remediable causes.

Admit if:

- The patient lives alone
- The patient will be left unsupervised for any duration of time
- If carers (or residential home) are unprepared/unable to continue looking after the patient *and/or*
- If history and examination have indicated a cause requiring acute hospital treatment, admit as an emergency.

Possible investigations to consider in the community

- Urine—dipstick for glucose, ketones, blood, protein, nitrates and white cells, send for M,C&S
- BM to exclude hypoglycaemia
- Blood—FBC, ESR, U&E, LFTs, TFTs
- ECG
- CXR.

Management at home
- Acute confusion is frightening for carers—reassure and support them.
- Treat the cause, e.g. antibiotics for UTI or chest infection.
- Try to avoid sedation as this can make confusion worse. Where unavoidable use haloperidol 1–2 mg prn or lorazepam 0.5–1 mg prn.
- Involve district nursing services, e.g. to provide incontinence aids, cot sides, moral support.
- If the cause does not become clear despite investigation or the patient fails to improve with treatment admit for further investigation and assessment.

Table 15.1 Causes of acute confusion

Infection	Particularly UTI, pneumonia; rarely encephalitis, meningitis
Drugs	Opiates, sedatives, L-dopa, anticonvulsants, recreational drugs
Metabolic	Hypoglycaemia, uraemia, liver failure, hypercalcaemia, other electrolyte imbalance (rarer)
Alcohol or drug withdrawal	
Hypoxia	e.g. severe pneumonia, exacerbation of COPD, cardiac failure
Cardiovascular	MI, stroke, TIA
Intracranial	Space occupying lesion, raised intracranial pressure, head injury (especially subdural haematoma)
Thyroid disease	Hyper- or hypothyroidism
Carcinomatosis	
Epilepsy	Temporal lobe epilepsy, post-ictal state
Nutritional deficiency	B_{12}, thiamine or nicotinic acid deficiency

⊛ Compulsory admission and treatment of patients with mental illness

Most requiring inpatient care for mental disorder agree to hospital admission and become 'informal' patients. A minority (~5%) require compulsory admission and detention under the Mental Health Act of 1983* and are termed 'Sectioned'—in reference to the Section of the Mental Health Act under which they are detained (Figure 15.3).

Procedure for 'sectioning' a patient

Applications can be made for:
- Admission for assessment under Section 2 (📖 p.261)
- Admission for treatment under Section 3 (📖 p.261)
- Emergency admission under Section 4 (📖 p.261)
- Guardianship under Section 7 (📖 p.261).

Applications can be made by:
- An approved social worker (ASW)
- The nearest relative of the person concerned. Nearest relative is defined in the Act as the 1st surviving person out of:
  - spouse (or co-habitee for >6 mo)
  - oldest child (if >18 y)
  - parent
  - oldest sibling (if >18 y)
  - grandparent
  - grandchild (>18 y)
  - uncle or aunt (>18 y)
  - nephew or niece (>18 y)
  - non-relative living with patient for ≥5 y.

The applicant (ASW or nearest relative) must have seen the patient <2wk (<24 h in the case of Section 4) before the date of the application.

❶ The ASW should be chosen rather than the nearest relative wherever possible, to avoid affecting family relationships.

Applications must be based on:
- 2 medical recommendations (except Section 4, which only needs 1). Doctors may examine the patient together or separately, but there must be <6 d between examinations. Recommendations must be signed on or before the date of application.
- Where 2 medical recommendations are required, the doctors should not be from the same hospital or practice *and* one of the doctors must be 'approved' under the Mental Health Act.
- One doctor, if practicable, must have prior knowledge of the patient (ideally a GP—but GPs are not obliged to attend outside the practice area). If neither doctor has prior knowledge of the patient, the applicant must state on the application why this was so.
- Medical recommendation(s) and application must concur on at least one form of mental disorder.

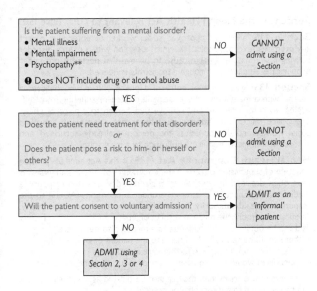

In practice 'Sectioning' means calling in the duty social worker and duty psychiatrist. It can be a time consuming and frustrating business. Always try to obtain voluntary admission—it is better for you and the patient.

Keep a supply of forms you might need for Sectioning—Forms 3, 7 and 10 (GP recommendation for Section 2, 4 and 3 respectively) and Form 5 (Application for Section 4 for a 'nearest relative') Deputizing doctors should always try and contact the patient's own GP.

Notes:

*   Applies in England and Wales only. In Northern Ireland similar provisions apply under the Mental Health (Northern Ireland) Order 1986. Scotland—see 📖 p.260

** Personality disorder characterized by inability to make loving relationships, antisocial behaviour and lack of guilt

Fig. 15.3 Deciding whether a 'Section' is needed.

❶ The Mental Health Act only allows for compulsory assessment and treatment of a patient's mental health problems—the patient may refuse consent for investigation and/or treatment of other health problems while 'sectioned'.

Sections of the Mental Health Act relevant to GPs: Table 15.2.

Section 115: allows an approved social worker to enter and inspect any premises (except hospital) in which a person with a mental disorder is living if s/he has reasonable cause to believe that person is not under proper care. Application through a magistrate is needed.

Section 135: gives right of entry of a police officer who believes a person with a mental disorder is being ill-treated or suffering from self-neglect to enter premises and remove that person to a place of safety. The police officer who attends must be accompanied by an approved social worker and doctor unless the person is already 'sectioned' and absent without leave. Requires application to a magistrate.

Mental Health Community Act (1995): this Act aims to 'provide a system of supervision of care in the community of certain patients who have been detained in hospital'. In England and Wales, the responsible medical officer applies for 'after-care under supervision' (ACUS) to the responsible health authority 6-monthly for the first year then yearly. Application can only be made in respect of a patient (≥16 y old) currently liable to be detained in hospital due to a mental disorder where:
- there could be serious risk of harm to the patient or others if the patient were not to receive further care services *and*
- supervision would help to ensure receipt of further care services.

If patients refuse treatment, they cannot be treated against their will but can be conveyed to a day centre or hospital.

Scotland: The Mental Health Act (Care and Treatment) (Scotland) 2003 provides for compulsory admission under Part 5 for 72 h. The application is made by a fully registered medical practitioner in consultation with a mental health officer, unless this is impracticable. In hospital Part 6 (lasting 28 d) can be applied and then, if necessary, Part 7 (Compulsory Treatment Order) for 6 mo.

Further information: ▣ www.scotland.gov.uk

Essential reading

Hyperguide to the Mental Health Act ▣ www.hyperguide.co.uk/mha

Table 15.2 Sections of the Mental Health Act relevant to primary care

Section	Notes	Application
Section 2: *Admission for assessment:*	Most commonly used section in the community. Admission for 28 d for assessment. Not renewable after that time. Patients may appeal within 2 wk of detention via the Mental Health Tribunal.	Application must be made by the nearest relative or an ASW on the recommendation of 2 doctors—one approved, and the other who has prior knowledge of the patient. If application is made by the ASW, the nearest relative should be informed before application or as soon as possible afterwards. Application is valid for 14 d.
Section 3: *Admission for treatment:*	Admission for treatment for ≤6 mo. The exact mental disorder must be stated. Detention is renewable for a further 6 mo and annually thereafter	Application must be made by the nearest relative or an ASW on the recommendation of 2 doctors—one approved, and the other who has prior knowledge of the patient. Application is valid for 14 d.
Section 4: *Emergency admission for assessment:*	Used in situations where admission is urgent and compliance with Section 2 would cause undesirable delay Admission to hospital for 72 h only. Not renewable. Usually converted to a Section 2 on arrival at hospital.	Application must be made by the nearest relative or an ASW. If application is made by the ASW, the nearest relative should be informed before application or as soon as possible afterwards. Medical recommendation is from *either* an approved doctor *or* a doctor with prior knowledge of the patient. Application is only valid for 24 h.
Section 7: *Guardianship*	A Guardian has power to: • require a person to live at a particular place • require a person to go to specific places at specific times for medical treatment, work, education or training • require a doctor, ASW or other specified person be given access to the person under Guardianship. ❶ Guardians can insist a person sees a doctor but cannot force treatment.	Application must be made by the nearest relative or an ASW on the recommendation of 2 doctors—one approved, and the other who has prior knowledge of the patient. Application is valid for 14 d.

Miscellaneous emergencies

Miscellaneous emergencies

⊛ **Sickle cell anaemia:** most common among people originating from areas in which malaria is endemic. Due to altered types of haemoglobin. Patients typically have a low Hb level (typically 8–9 g/dl) but compensate well. Consider all patients to be hyposplenic.

Management of acute illness
- Maintain adequate hydration.
- Treat infection early (infection is the commonest cause of death).
- Give analgesia for painful crises—admit if severe.
- Admit if significant crisis of any sort (e.g. stroke, dyspnoea, acute abdomen, aplastic anaemia).

⌂ **Haemophilia and other clotting factor deficiencies:**

Clinical features: bleeding → joints or muscles is often delayed following trauma. If untreated, results in permanent damage. Pressure effects occur if bleeding takes place into a confined space, e.g. intracranial bleed. Severity of bleeding is related to levels of clotting factors.

Management: treatment can be 'on demand' or 'prophylactic'. All haemophiliacs should have long-term follow-up via a specialist haemophilia centre.

On-demand treatment
- Transfusion of factor VIII or IX preparation as soon as possible after bleeding has started—most administer it to themselves
- Symptomatic treatment of bleeds, e.g. rest, analgesia ± physiotherapy for bleeds in muscles/joints.

Prophylactic treatment: prevents bleeds and their consequences. Tranexamic acid, desmopressin or specific clotting factors.

⊛ **Acute jaundice** yellow pigmentation due to excess bile pigment (clinical jaundice when serum bilirubin >35 µmol/l). May be pre-hepatic (due to haemolysis), hepatic (hepatitis, cirrhosis) or post-hepatic (obstructive due to carcinoma, gallstones, sepsis, primary sclerosing cholangitis). All jaundice needs investigating to establish a cause, if unwell or rapidly progressive -admit, else refer for urgent out-patient appointment.

⌂ **Liver failure:** presents with sudden onset of severe illness.

Features: ≥1 of:
- Jaundice
- Hypoglycaemia
- Hepatic encephalopathy (ranges from mild confusion and irritability through drowsiness and increasing confusion to coma)
- Haemorrhage—due to deranged clotting factors
- Infection
- Ascites—hepatosplenomegaly and ascites are not usually prominent.

Management: admit as emergency to a hepatologist/gastroenterologist unless an expected terminal event. Prognosis is poor (<60% survive).

⚙ **Wound dehiscence:** Breakdown of a surgical wound – usually abdominal. May be partial or complete. Readmit for further assessment except if very minor—when refer for urgent out-patient review. If complete dehiscence, cover with a sterile pack soaked in saline.

◉ **Acute intermittent porphyria:** Rare, inherited metabolic disorder. Porphyrins are important in the manufacture of haemoglobin. Deficiency of enzymes in the porphyrin pathway results in build up of intermediary which are toxic to skin and nervous system.

Presentation: fever, GI symptoms (vomiting, abdominal pain – can be severe); neuropsychiatric symptoms (hypotonia, paralysis, fits, impaired vision, peripheral neuritis, odd behaviour – even psychosis). Urine may go deep red on standing.

Management: Specialist management is required. Advise avoidance of precipitants. Treat acute attacks symptomatically.

☺ Confirmation and certification of death

⚠ The death certification process in England and Wales is currently under review and likely to change in the near future.

English law *does not* require a doctor
- To confirm death has occurred or that 'life is extinct'. A doctor is only required to certify what, in their opinion, was the cause;
- To view the body of a deceased person. There is no obligation to see/examine a body before issuing a death certificate;
- to report the fact that death has occurred.

English law *does* require the doctor who attended the deceased during the last illness to issue a certificate detailing the cause of death. Certificates are provided by the local Registrar of births, marriages and deaths. A special certificate is needed for infants of <28 d old.

Death in the community: ¼ occur at home.

Expected deaths: in all cases, advise to contact the undertakers and ensure the patient's own GP is notified.
- *Patient's home:* visit as soon as practicable.
- *Residential/nursing home:* if possible the GP who attended during the patient's last illness should visit and issue a death certificate. The 'on-call' GP is often requested to visit. There is no statutory duty to do this but it is reassuring for the staff at the home and often necessary before staff are allowed to ask for the body to be removed.

Unexpected and/or 'sudden' death: if called, advise the attendant to call 999. Visit and take a rapid history from any attendants. Then:
- *Resuscitate if appropriate*—drowning and hypothermia can protect against hypoxic neurological damage; brains of children <5y. old are more resistant to damage.
- *Report the death to the coroner*—If any suspicious circumstances or circumstances of death are unknown/unclear—call the police.

Alternatively if police or ambulance service is already in attendance and death has been confirmed, suggest the police surgeon is contacted.

Cremation: The Cremation Acts of 1902 and 1952 require 2 doctors to complete a certificate to establish identity and that the cause of death is not suspicious before a person can be cremated. A fee is payable to each doctor by the person arranging the funeral. It has 2 parts:
- *Part B:* completed by the patient's usual medical attendant—usually his/her GP.
- *Part C:* completed by another doctor who must have held full GMC registration (or equivalent) for ≥5 y and is not connected with the patient in any way nor directly connected with the doctor who issued part B—usually a GP from another practice.

⚠ Pacemakers and radioactive implants must be removed from the deceased before cremation can take place.

Further information on completing cremation forms
Home Office 🖳 www.dca.gov.uk/corbur/cremation_forms_guidance.pdf

> **Box 16.1 Deaths that must be reported to the coroner**
> - Sudden or unexpected deaths
> - Accidents and injuries
> - Industrial diseases, e.g. mesothelioma
> - Service disability pensioners
> - Deaths where the doctor has not attended within the past 14 d
> - Deaths arising from ill treatment, e.g. abuse, neglect, starvation, hypothermia
> - Cause of death unknown
> - Deaths <24 h. After hospital admission
> - Poisoning (chronic alcoholism and its sequelae are no longer notifiable)
> - Medical mishaps (including anaesthetic complications, short- or long-term complications of operations, drugs—whether therapeutic or addictive)
> - Abortions
> - Prisoners
> - Stillbirths (if there is doubt about whether the baby was born alive)

Notification of death to the coroner: the coroner can be contacted via the local police. Reporting to the coroner does not automatically entail a post mortem. The coroner, once circumstances of death are clear, may advise the GP to tick and initial box A on the back of the certificate which advises the Registrar that no inquest is necessary. Deaths which *MUST* be reported to the coroner are listed in Box 16.1.

❶ In Scotland deaths are reported to a procurator fiscal. The list of reportable deaths is the same with the addition of deaths of foster children and the newborn.

Recording deaths in primary care: death registers are useful. Routine communication of deaths to all members of the primary healthcare team and other agencies involved with the care of that patient (e.g. hospital consultants, social services) avoids the embarrassing and distressing situation of ongoing appointments and contacts being made for that patient. Record the death in the notes of any relatives/partner registered with the practice.

Patient advice and support

Department of work and pensions (DWP) Leaflet D49: What to do after a death in England and Wales. Available from 🖥 www.dwp.gov.uk

Scottish Executive What to do after a death in Scotland. Available from 🖥 www.scotland.gov.uk

Office of Fair Trading. Arranging funerals. 🖥 www.direct.gov.uk

Index

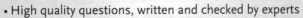